THE COMMUNICATION OF CARING IN NURSING

BY VIRGINIA KNOWLDEN, RN, EdD

SIGMA THETA TAU INTERNATIONAL
CENTER NURSING PRESS
PEER-REVIEWED PUBLICATIONS

Date	Title
1992	Leonard Felix Fuld, 19th Century Reformer in the 20th Century World
1997	The Image Editors: Mind, Spirit, and Voice
1997	The Language of Nursing Theory and Metatheory
1997	The Adventurous Years: Leaders in Action, 1973-1993, a Nell Watts Memoir
1997	Virginia Avenel Henderson: Signature for Nursing
1998	The Neuman Systems Model and Nursing Education: Teaching Strategies and Outcomes
1998	Immigrant Women and Their Health: An Olive Paper

For other Center Nursing Press publications and videos contact:
Sigma Theta Tau International
550 West North Street
Indianapolis, IN 46202
1.888.634.7575
FAX: 317.634.8188
www.stti.iupui.edu

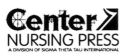

ISBN: 0-9656391-7-7

Printed in the United States of America.

Table of Contents

LIST OF TABLES AND FIGURES

Acknowledgements

THANKS TO:

June Brodie and Eugene Martin at Columbia University,
Teachers College and the Lindbergh Foundation,
who set me on the path.

All the nurses and patients who participated
unstintingly in these studies.

Members of the St. Joseph College Qualitative
Research Circle, especially Esther, Helen R., and Nancy,
who kept me on the path.

Nursing students at St. Joseph College who contributed to the
development of the theory.

And, especially, my family particularly Gail, Lyn, and Alex—
for being.

Chapter 1

INTRODUCTION

"You ... Feel Caring Through ... Touch ... [And Speech]"

(Knowlden, 1985, p. 111)

Caring is a universal human phenomenon. It is widely acknowledged to be essential for the growth of human beings. The presence of caring among people evokes particular behaviors in every culture. Caring has in the past assisted in the continued survival of humans and continues to play an essential part in the evolution of humankind. The meaning of caring is interpreted from the behaviors that arise from a particular culture's social expectations about its people and which are approved and rewarded as such.

My interest in and concern about caring arose while leading post-clinical conferences in an urban hospital school of nursing with senior nursing students who were learning in an intensive care unit (ICU). Our discussions focused on the psychosocial aspects of providing nursing care to their patients.

The number of experiences the students had that they described as "overwhelming" was outstanding. How can students provide caring to patients if they are overwhelmed by their working environment? The topic for one of the conferences, "How do you provide caring to patients despite the tubes and technology?," led to the question that was asked in the second of the two studies presented in this monograph.

In the first study, *The Meaning of Caring in the Nursing Role* (Knowlden, 1985), nurses and patients were asked to indicate from a videotape of a nurse-patient home care situation what they saw that indicated caring. In the second study, *Caring in Nursing: Is it Surviving in High-tech Settings?* (1988), nurses and patients or parents of patients in intensive care settings were asked how the nurse got beyond tubes and technology to provide caring. It would seem intuitively obvious that caring is essential to nursing. Yet there have been few empirical studies of caring published in nursing literature.

In this monograph, I explore and extend the meaning of caring derived from the experiences of patients and nurses in actual nursing situations. This monograph represents another step toward knowledge of caring in nursing drawn from interpretations of caring based on empirical data. It describes nurses' experiences with patients and their problems, and patients' experiences with nurses and nursing care. These studies of caring in nurse-patient relationships address the real world of nursing and have the potential to contribute to progress in nursing science. The studies were focused on the meaning of caring in nursing situations through the actions of nurses as gathered from the perceptions of both nurses and patients.

The study of caring in nursing is the study of a concept generally held to be important for nursing (Benner, 1984; Bevis, 1982; Leininger, 1977; Roach, 1984; Watson, 1979). Studying caring acknowledges the value and the importance of the meaning of the interpersonal relationship that occurs between the patient and the nurse attending to the patient's health. Studying caring reflects nurses' concern for the well-being of others.

Above all, the study of caring contributes to the goal of nursing which, as an art and a science, is to promote optimal health and self-actualization in human beings through protective, nurturing, and generative activities. Nursing actions are intended to provide assistance and support through the patient's intrapersonal, interpersonal, and community systems to facilitate health. Community in this instance means the personal support of family, friends, and relatives—as well as the network of agency representatives that provide health care to people in need.

The study of the meaning of caring is presented in a thorough, organized, and systematic manner for the development of the discipline of nursing. Published studies of caring can help readers explore "what happens in caring situations, and (predicted) future caring encounters" (Leininger, 1980, p. 135).

Caring is a basic philosophic concern of nursing practice. Nurses attempt to cure through care and treatment (Merriam-Webster, 1995). Indeed, healing in nursing is based on care and treatment. Leininger (1977) believes that "caring is the essence and central focus of nursing ... decisions, practice, and goals" (p. 2). Caring refers to those aspects of nursing that are intrinsic to actual nurse-patient processes that produce therapeutic results in patients (Watson, 1979).

Organizing nursing around processes identified as caring places the practice of nursing in its proper perspective. When caring is perceived as the central focus in nursing—the patient, demands, skills, expectations, and self-congruence in the nursing role are balanced.

Caring is like a fulcrum from which nursing care is provided. It is in caring for the patient that the dichotomy of tenderness and technique becomes integrated (Meyer, 1960). The knowledge and the skills of nurses are necessary so that patients may be healed.

The study of caring reveals patterns of human behavior as people interact in health-enhancing contexts. Studying caring enables the expression of the concern nurses have with the processes by which positive changes in health status are effected (Donaldson & Crowley, 1978). Caring attempts to create a relationship which will empower the growth of others as separate people. It provides the frame of reference for a nurse's practice.

HISTORY OF THE PROBLEM

To search for the meaning of caring in the practice of nursing is to search for the meaning of a fundamental expectation society holds for the nursing profession. Yet caring has been increasingly displaced by the economics, technology, and mechanization of health care—and by the concomitant depersonalization of patients and nurses. Nursing and nursing care have been positively and negatively affected by the industrialization and bureaucratization of society.

A contemporary concern expressed by nurse clinicians, theorists, and educators is that some nurses do not treat patients as people, but instead treat them as objects to which certain skills are applied. Thus some raise the question of whether nurses care for patients or for machines and systems.

Health care in recent decades has increasingly adapted to the proliferation of mechanical equipment, computer technology, and pressures of health care economics. As a consequence, nurse-patient relationships have been obscured through introduction of mechanical objects and organizational systems that intervene between nurses and patients. Patients may experience a loss of identity by being treated as an object instead of a person and from being perceived abstractly as a component of some amorphous context (Drew, 1986). Patients often have minimal opportunity to affect the interaction because they are subjected to a type of health care that tends to depersonalize both patients and nurses. The specialization and institutionalization of health care and the reductionistic development of science have contributed to depersonalized care. Contributions made by medicoscientific discoveries and technologies can overshadow individual patients, reduce patients to "objects," and become tyrannical agents untempered by a humanistic value system (Carper, 1979).

Nurses promote health through interpersonal processes as well as through technologic activities—both therapeutic in purpose. Nurses obtain direction from this focus on human capacities and strengths (Bevis, 1981). Nurses' actions are carried out in a therapeutic alliance in which nurses and patients are joined. The results are caring actions determined by nurses and patients to improve patients' health. However, if nurses perceive patients as objects toward which certain actions are directed, this therapeutic alliance will not materialize. While patients might receive treatment, the persons will not be cared for. It is this concern about the possibility of nurses depersonalizing patients and other nurses which drives the contemporary research about caring in nursing.

CONCEPTUAL FRAMEWORK

Concern about the meaning that nurses' actions had to both patients and nurses influenced the studies from the perspectives of symbolic interactionism and philosophy of caring.

SYMBOLIC INTERACTIONISM

Symbolic interactionism has the potential for framing questions concerning the phenomenon of caring in nursing. One of the many role theories, symbolic interactionism was developed by George Herbert Mead and promulgated by his followers from the Chicago School, as the University of Chicago's Sociology Department was known in the 1920s, notably Herbert Blumer. Symbolic interactionism followers investigate reciprocal social relations and emphasize the significance of self-reflection in actions between people.

Symbolic interactionism holds that the human mind, the notion of the social self, and the structures in society all emerge through reciprocal social interactions (Hardy & Hardy, 1988). It focuses on the meaning that the social acts and the symbols of the actors in the process of interaction have for each other (Hardy, 1988). "Actor(s) tend ... to construct a given situation as it seems to [them] ... [in the] definition of the situation.... It is on the basis of each actor's definition that subsequent actions take place" (Conway, 1978, p. 68).

As Blumer (1969) states,

The human being is not a mere responding organism only responding to the play of factors from his world or from himself; he is an acting organism who has to cope with and handle such factors and who in so doing has to forge and direct his line of action (p. 55).

Symbolic interactionism is grounded in three premises:
- human beings act toward things on the basis of the meanings that the things have for them;
- the meanings of the things are derived from, or arise out of, the social interaction one has with one's fellows;
- these meanings are handled in, and modified through, an interpretative process used by the person in dealing with the things encountered. (Blumer, 1969, p. 2)

Prus (1996), in his recent text on symbolic interaction, adds these seven assumptions about human group life: It is (a) intersubjective, (b) multi perspectiv[al], (c) reflective, (d) activity-based, (e) negotiable, (f) relational, (g) processual (pp. 15-18). He notes that

the primary conceptual and methodologic implication of this processual emphasis is that because all aspects of group life take place in process terms or take their shape over time, *it is essential that the human condition be conceptualized and studied in ways acutely mindful of the emergent nature of human lived experience.* (pp. 17-18).

The theory of symbolic interactionism begins with human beings in a cooperating group. Individuals' acts are explained through society, the organized complex conduct of that group.

The probable beginning of human communication was in coopera-tion ... where conduct differed and yet where the act of the one answered to and called out the act of the other.... [H]ere we have ... the medium of communication and reflection. (G.H. Mead [1909] as cited in Joas, 1985, p. 100)

Thus, intersubjectivity occurs between people as the result of a struc-ture of communicative relations between them which goes beyond the individual. Through intersubjectivity, the joint actions of people achieve life's needs (Joas, 1985).

For ... the whole (society) is prior to the part (the individual), not the part to the whole; and the part is explained in terms of the whole, not the whole in terms of the part of parts. (Mead, G.H., 1934, p. 7)

Meaning also arises out of intersubjectivity. For it is only when two or more people act together that meaning can occur. Out of the intentional act of one person through communication, meaning is conveyed to an-other. This is not to say that meaning is not also conveyed intrasubjectively when a person thinks about something. "Meaning is the consciousness of the relation between one's own actions and the responses of the other to them, which one can anticipate" (Joas, 1985, p. 105). Mead (1956) in his discussion of meaning indicated,

For the nature of meaning ... is found to be implicit in the structure of the social act, implicit in the relations among its three basic indi-vidual components: namely, in the triadic relation of a gesture of one individual, a response to that gesture by a second individual, and completion of the given social act initiated by the gesture of the first individual. And the fact that the nature of meaning is thus found to be implicit in the structure of a social act provides additional empha-sis upon the necessity ... of starting with the initial assumption of an ongoing social process of experience and behavior in which any given group of human individuals is involved, and upon which the exist-ence and development of their minds, selves, and self-consciousness depend. (p. 168)

But human relations are more than coordinated communication. Human relations are more than the sere structure of gesture, response gesture, and return gesture. Within these gestures are communicated the meaning which we as humans infer from the other's action in that situation. It is from these inferences that we come to know who we are as humans, how others are as humans, and how we are together as humans. Knowing another gives meaning to life. And for nursing, that meaning is caring for or about other humans in need.

PHILOSOPHERS ON CARING

From the writings of the philosopher Mayeroff (1971), we can sense that the therapeutic alliance between nurses and patients enable nurses to gain information about who a patient is in the world, the difficulties that are being experienced, and the collaboration that is possible between them for the patient's health. Nurses step back from nursing care actions to see what these actions amount to, and to maintain or change behaviors to better assist patients toward health. Even though nurses take account for the past in providing care, nursing care is provided in the here-and-now. Nurses know that it is in the present moment only that they are in control and can have an influence on the future health of the patient.

Behaviors that nurses use are guided by history, the meaning of past and present events, and insight from the past—while simultaneously the present moment is enriched by anticipation of the future. Using caring actions, nurses are enabled to understand patients and their personal world, because nurses are "inside" it. Such understanding enables patients to not feel alone, to believe they are understood, to be open—allowing nurses to be close in that world, not just knowing patients from the outside. These inclusive nursing actions toward patients permit both to "be-in-place" (Mayeroff, 1971).

Being-in-place is finding and making our place in the world so that the person who finds the self has helped to create that self. Being-in-place is the change that occurs in a human's life when that person comes to take full responsibility for that life. Being-in-place is both temporal and spatial and involves compatibility and harmony (Mayeroff, 1971). Caring gives meaning to nursing, and the goal of caring reflects the concept of the primacy of one person's relationship to another (Knowlden, 1983, unpublished paper). The examination of caring in nursing acknowledges the importance of the relationship between a patient and nurse. It reflects a nurse's concern for the well-being of others as a primary aspect of an interpersonal relationship.

Gabriel Marcel (1951) is also concerned with relatedness between people. He sees the world as a "broken world," a world divided between science, bureaucracies, and denial of self; and another world which affirms self (Marcel, 1951).

In the first world, body and mind are separate; feeling does not belong to the self. Experience is encrusted such that meaning is obscured. Realities are not represented to the self. Compartmentalization of experience prevents the self from responding to the novelty of experience. Thicker and thicker screens are interposed between the self and existence. This first world dissolves the unity of experience. Here attempts are made to scientifically categorize all lived experiences (Marcel, 1951).

In the second world, the unity of experience is rejoined. My body is felt as my body. It is no longer an instrument, an object. There is an "exclamatory awareness of self." The self is seen as an "existential indubitable" (Marcel, 1951). Experience is not just a passive recording of impressions, but an active, mindful relationship between perceptions, understanding, and the facts of the experience themselves. The self is separate from the world, but gains its particularity only in connection with and in apposition to an infinite number of other selves, other somebodies. Marcel believes this connection with others allows our reason to be led by the appearance of them. Our understanding is formed from others' presentation of themselves. The other is placed centrally so that something appears. This something then crosses a domain open to our encounter (Marcel, 1951).

A theologian, Martin Buber, has also written about human relationships between the self and others. The drive toward relation is primary. Although his words differ from the philosophers Mayeroff and Marcel, Buber (1970) stated,

> Man becomes an I through a You. What confronts us comes and vanishes, relational events take shape and scatter, and through these changes crystallizes, more and more each time, the consciousness of the constant partner, the I-consciousness. (p. 80)

Here, too, is that knowledge that the I, the self, is able to be both separate and joined with the other. Buber has a marvelous capacity to enable the reader to understand this I-It:I-You relationship:

> The unlimited sway of causality in the It-world, which is of fundamental importance for the scientific ordering of nature, is not felt to be oppressive by the man who is not confined to the It-world but free to step out of it again and again into the world of relation. Here I and You confront each other freely in a reciprocity that is not involved in or tainted by any causality; here man finds guaranteed the freedom of his being and of being. Only those who know relation and who know of the present of the You have the capacity for decision. (p. 100)

Without caring, humans are unable to survive, to develop, to self-actualize, to relate humanly. Without caring, humankind cannot survive. Through caring for certain specific others, by serving others through caring, some people live the meaning of their own lives.

NURSE THEORISTS ON CARING

The major writers about caring in nursing provide thoughtful comments about this philosophic idea. For Leininger, "Caring is the essence of nursing...." (1977, p. 2). For Roach (1984),

[C]aring is the human mode of being.... [N]ursing is the professionalization of human caring through deliberate affirmation of caring as the human mode of being and through the calling forth of the capacity or power to care through the acquisition of knowledge and expertise—cognitive, affective, technical, administrative skills specific to the practice of nursing as a helping discipline. (p. 1) Professionalization of human caring in nursing also takes into account the significance of caring as responsivity—caring as response to value. (p. 13) Professional caring is of the nature of a deliberate response to "that which matters," the important-in-itself, involving the spiritual power of affectivity. (p. 18)

Watson (1988) states, "Caring is presented as a moral ideal of nursing with a concern for preservation of humanity, dignity and the fullness of self." For Benner and Wrubel (1989), "Caring ... means that persons, events, projects, and things matter to people." Benner and Wrubel base their work on the premise that "an articulation of alternative approaches to health promotion, restoration, and even curing practices [are] based upon the primacy of caring." Bishop and Scudder (1991) hold that nursing is the practice of caring "with an inherent moral sense" (p. 18). "The dominant sense in nursing practice" (1990, p. 173).

The moral sense is actually realized through a personal relationship between nurses and patients. This personal relation has three dominant senses: the first calls for establishing a dialogical relation which is triadic since the relation has an end beyond itself; the second for treating the patient with the dignity and worth due a person; and the third for expressing through nursing practice every nurse's personal response to a particular patient. (1990, p. 175)

Bishop and Scudder "believe that the philosophy of nursing, when appropriately developed, actually becomes a philosophy of practice" (1990, p. 9). They find that "in practice, nursing ethics is based primarily on trust and mutuality" (1990, p. 11). "As a result, nursing holds a privileged position ... between physicians, patients, themselves, and hospital bureaucrats ... from which to make moral decisions concerning patient care" (1990, pp. 10-11). Bishop and Scudder say that their beliefs "should speak forcefully to those nurses who have a deep appreciation for the caring tradition" (1990, p. 11).

NURSE RESEARCHERS ON CARING

In the last two decades, interest about caring in nursing has grown. This interest has been manifested in the proliferation of essays and research on the subject. Several attempts have been made to analyze the research findings (Andrews, Daniels, & Hull, 1996; Lea & Watson, 1996; Morse, Bottorff, Neander, & Solberg, 1991; Morse, Solberg, Neander, Bottorff, & Johnson, 1990; Warren, 1988). Of these, the two reviews by Morse and colleagues are the most comprehensive and comprehensible.

Morse and colleagues (1990, 1991) indicate that caring is a diffuse and elusive concept. Kaplan (1964) noted that some conceptions have a family of meanings, so that no fixed definition may be possible. Rather, features are shared and the meaning of a word "is a family affair among its senses" (p. 48). Just as conceptualizations change with use, so do concepts. "Both may be viewed either in terms of what is in fact at work to fulfill the purposes of [the] process...." (Kaplan, p. 49). Caring is one such concept that appears to consist of a family of meanings. Yet, as Morse and colleagues make evident, for caring theory to be of use to the nursing profession and its practice, the various conceptualizations require thorough explication and exploration of the derivative. Shiber and Larson (1991) also direct attention to the delineation of patient outcomes that occur as the result of the process of nursing caring and its structural components.

Morse and colleagues (1990, 1991), drawing from the writings of 35 nurse theorists, identified five conceptualizations of caring: as a human trait, as a moral imperative or ideal, as an affect, as an interpersonal relationship, and as a therapeutic intervention. They also identified three outcomes (1991): patients' subjective and physical responses, and nurses' subjective experience. They concluded that "the first desperately needed step is to develop a clear conceptualization of caring that encompasses all aspects of nursing ... [and] the focus of theory and research must shift to incorporate a focus on the patient" (Morse et al., 1990).

Valentine (1989a, 1989b, 1989c, 1991) has attempted through her research to relate caring to outcome measures. She conducted her study in a hospital setting with matched pairs of 91 hysterectomy patients and their nurses (1989b), and considered the relevant "context, resources, processes, and outcomes" (1991, p. 59). She used qualitative and quantitative research methods organized through application of a decision-oriented evaluation framework–the Stufflebeam context-input-process-product (CIPP) model as cited in Valentine, 1991. Use of this model required having different samples of participants and data collection procedures during its four phases.

The following two researchers' studies are included in this brief review because both nurses and patients were participants in the studies. This is important in response to Morse and colleagues and Shiber and Larson's recommendation and because it is an important feature of this monograph. Although there has been much research concerning caring in nursing, some investigators have had only nurses or patients as research participants.

From her studies concerning perinatal nursing, Swanson (1986, 1991, 1993) has developed a middle-range theory of caring. Five caring processes were explicated from this series of phenomenologic studies—knowing, being with, doing for, enabling, and maintaining belief. Swanson also provides a definition of caring as "a nurturing way of relating to a valued other toward whom one feels a personal sense of commitment and responsibility" (1991, p. 165). She contrasts nurse caring with social support and notes that social support implies a mutual obligation between caregiver and receiver. In nursing, no such mutual obligation is intended: "The nurse cares without obligating the client to reciprocate" (1991, p. 165). Linkages are made to Watson's transpersonal nurse caring theory (1985) and Benner's (1984) research concerning the helping role of nurses. Swanson contends that "caring is a central and unifying nursing phenomenon; it does not, however, render the concept of caring as unique to nursing knowledge or practice" (1991, p. 165).

In 1993, Swanson presented her theory of caring as a structure of caring which "linked ... the nurses' philosophic attitude, informed understandings, message conveyed, therapeutic actions, and intended outcome" (p. 355). Swanson "depicts caring as grounded in maintenance of a basic belief in person, anchored in knowing the other's reality, conveyed through being with, and enacted through doing for and enabling" (p. 357).

The use by Wolf, Giardino, Osborne, and Ambrose (1994) of Wolf's Caring Behaviors Inventory (CBI) revised, revealed a five-factor solution for the 43-item instrument. The five factors, dimensions of nursing caring, were respectful deference to others, assurance of human presence, positive connectedness, professional knowledge and skill, and attentiveness to the other's experience. A convenience sample of 278 nurses and 263 patients from secondary or tertiary health care settings participated in the study.

The CBI researchers had established test-retest reliability with a nurse sample. Internal consistency reliability of 0.96 alpha coefficient resulted from the combined nurse-patient sample. Construct validity of contrasted group types was also established on the total scores of both groups. Wolf and colleagues note that this is a preliminary study with several limitations related to sampling method, sample size, instrumentation, and reliability and validity. However, the authors suggest that the factors generated by the revised CBI relate to Watson's (1988) Transpersonal Caring Theory.

In summary, absence of uniformity continues among the conceptualizations of nursing caring. Despite the numbers of studies reported, few present both nurses' and patients' perceptions of nurse caring. Overlapping evidence of congruence exists between the Swanson study and that of Wolf and colleagues. This is demonstrated in the parallel titles of being with (Swanson, 1991)—assurance of human presence and positive connectedness (Wolf et al., 1994), and knowing (Swanson)—professional knowledge and skill (Wolf et al.). However, no parallels are apparent for doing for, enabling, and maintaining belief (Swanson), or for respectful deference to others, and attentiveness to the other's experience (Wolf et al.).

In this monograph, I address several of the lacunae in nurse caring research that Morse and colleagues and Shiber and Larson indicated. The conceptualization of nurse caring is based on empirical data and inductive reasoning instead of the speculation, conceptualization, and deductive reasoning that comprises much of the research in this area. Caring has been viewed interactionally—not merely from the perspective of only the nurse or only the patient. Meanings of caring are analyzed in two almost diametrically opposed contexts of nursing care—in acute ICUs within hospitals, and in home care. As a result, the data obtained are extremely rich. The viewing and watching of videotaped nurse-patient encounters fit well with symbolic interactionist and grounded theory assumptions, an innovative approach about meanings in context and ascertaining symbolic meaning interactionally between researchers and patients or nurses.

A DEFINITION OF CARING

Upon initiating the original study (Knowlden, 1985), a conceptual analysis of caring drawn from a review of the literature then available was completed. The following definition was developed to guide the study:

Caring in nursing are those appropriate acts toward or for another individual or group who have evident or anticipated health needs. These acts occur in response to a feeling of concern and solicitude, and regard safety and well-being, ameliorate or improve a human condition, maintain charge or responsibility, provide for or attend to needs, or perform necessary services. Nursing acts include but are not limited to assisting, consulting, enabling, facilitating, generating, health consulting, health instructing, health promoting, nurturing, protecting, restoring, stimulating, and supporting. (p. 13)

As in any study in which interpretation of the data contributes to understanding a concept, at the conclusion of interpretation a second definition of caring emerged:

Caring is an interpersonal communication between nurse and patient. It consists of the irreducible aspects of content and relationship. Nursing content includes health teaching, assessment, physical care, advocacy, knowledge, supplying resources, planning for the future, and safety. Relationship aspects are concern, progress, and hope; listening; the personal relationship between the patient and nurse; building self-esteem; touching, laughter, and humor; being gentle and careful; telling what is found; being considerate, understanding, and collaborating; and counseling (Knowlden, 1985) (Figure 1.1).

After synthesis of the data from the two studies, interpretation led to a third definition of caring. Such a definition will be given later in the monograph.

In Chapter Two, I introduce information concerning the settings for the studies and the methods for data collection, analysis, and synthesis. In Chapter Three, I provide the synthesis of the findings; in Chapter Four, I discuss the conditions for caring. Conclusions are presented in Chapter Five and the substantiation of the research as a theory of caring in nursing in Chapter Six.

Figure 1.1 The Communication of Caring in Nursing (Model 1)

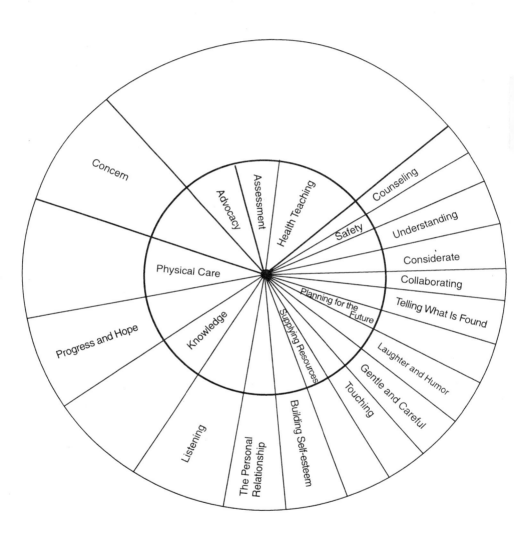

Inner Circle = Content
Outer Circle = Relationship

Chapter 2

EXPLORING THE MEANING OF CARING IN NURSING—SETTINGS AND METHODS

In this chapter the settings, contexts, and environments of the two studies, *The Meaning of Caring in the Nursing Role* and "Caring in Nursing: Is it Surviving in High-tech Health Settings?" are discussed. Brief demographic information about the studies and the methods of data collection and analysis are presented. In addition, similarities and differences between the two are noted.

SETTINGS

Settings for the two studies were quite different. The 1985 study in home-health settings was conducted in a populous Mid-Atlantic section of the United States and centered on nurses caring for patients in their homes. The nurses were employees of home-health agencies, and the patients were clients of these agencies. The participating nurses chose as research participants patients with whom they had worked for at least six visits, and from whom they had obtained verbal consent to participate in the research.

The home-health agencies were also quite different demographically. One agency was based in a hospital located in an old industrial city and the patients (and their parents, in the case of children) were referred from that hospital. The other two agencies were visiting nurse associations that received their referrals from agencies and physicians in the county. The hospital agency was in an inner city; the two visiting nurse associations were in suburban areas of cities that were county seats.

The 1988 study was about nurse caring in ICUs. This study was conducted in a southern New England state. The ICU nurses were employees of four hospitals. Three hospitals were in an inner city area; the other in a suburban area. The sites for participants' selection were cardiac, neonatal and pediatric (in which case parents were interviewed), and surgical ICUs. Nurses who volunteered to participate in the study provided the researcher with names of patients they had cared for in the ICUs. Verbal consent was obtained to participate in the research.

DEMOGRAPHIC DATA

In the home-health study, 33 patients participated; in the ICU study, 12 participated for a total of 45. Nineteen nurses participated in each study for a total of 38 nurse participants. Written consent to participate in the studies was obtained from all participants—or, in the case of infants and children, from parents—to assure that anonymity and confidentiality would be maintained. Participants in the home-health study were aware that the videotapes and interview materials were retained for research and education purposes, and in the ICU study, participants were informed that the interview materials were to be retained for research and education purposes.

PATIENTS' DEMOGRAPHIC DATA

In the study of caring in home-health settings, 12 of the patients were retired women with a chronic illness. Six were children under 3 years of age; their parents were present during the videotaping. Those parents who were available were interviewed for the second part of the data collection for this study. Six participants were between the ages of 3 and 59, and 21 participants were between the ages of 60 and 99. Fifteen of the adult participants were high school graduates, nine had completed post high school education. Six patients were ill with cancer and four with complications of diabetes.

Of the 12 patients in the ICU study, five were under 1 year of age and six were between age 51 and 80. Four of the participants had completed high school or college. The diagnosis of the five infants was prematurity. The adults had varying diagnoses.

The demographic data obtained in both studies were combined (Tables 2.1-2.5) and reviewed. The tables show the findings for both patient and nurse participants. When the combined patients' demographic data were reviewed, almost 25 percent of the patients were 1 year of age or younger, and slightly more than 25 percent were between 61 and 70 years of age. Most patient participants, however, were over 40 years of age ($N=30$, or 67%) and most had completed high school, college, or other higher education.

NURSES' DEMOGRAPHIC DATA

In the home health care study, the 19 nurses—all women—had at least baccalaureate degrees in nursing. Although 13 had diploma or associate degrees, one of these had completed the master's degree. Their average age was 28 years.

Table 2.1 Demographic Data: Patients		n=45
Age in Years	n	%
0-3	11	24
4-20	01	02
21-30	03	07
31-40	00	00
41-50	02	04
51-60	03	07
61-70	13	29
71-80	09	20
Over 80	03	07

Table 2.2 Demographic Data: Patients		n=45
Education	n	%
No formal education	11	24
(infants, preschoolers, adults)		
Grade school	06	13
High school	17	38
College/other higher education	11	24

Table 2.3 Demographic Data: Patients	n=45
Sex	n
Female	29
Male	16

Table 2.4 Demographic Data: Patients		n=45
Occupations	n	%
Accountant	01	02
Banker	01	02
Children	12	27
Educator	01	02
Export financier	01	02
Homemaker	12	27
Retired	10	22
Secretary, office worker	07	16

Table 2.5 Demographic Data: Patients	$n=45$
Diagnoses	n
Abdominal aortic aneurysm	01
Abscess of arm	01
Anorexia nervosa	01
Arthritis	03
Astrocytoma	01
Brachipalsy in infant	01
Cancer	06
Chronic obstructive pulmonary disease	01
Congestive heart failure	04
Cardiovascular accident	02
Diabetes with complications	04
Glioma	01
Hypertension with complications	02
Myocardial infarction	02
Multiple sclerosis	03
Obesity	01
Prematurity	06
Prematurity with twins	02
Pulmonary abscess	02

Eighteen of the nurses in the intensive care study were women and one was a man. Nine were between the ages of 20 and 29, and 10 were between 30 and 39. Eleven had graduated from baccalaureate programs as their basic nursing education preparation. Two of these had subsequently completed a master's degree in nursing. None of the nurses with either an associate degree or a diploma in nursing had completed baccalaureate degrees.

A review of the combined nurse participants' demographic data (Tables 2.6-2.7) showed that 33 were between 20 and 39 years of age, and six were between 40 and 59. Their basic educational preparation reflected the three levels of entry into registered nurse practice: associate degree, diploma, and baccalaureate degree. Initially 17 were educated in baccalaureate nursing programs; 21 were prepared in diploma or associate degree programs. Data presented in the category *Highest Degree Achieved* showed that 27 had baccalaureate degrees—although not all in nursing—and three had master's degrees in nursing.

Table 2.6 Demographic Data: Nurses		n=39
Age in Years	n	%
20-29	17	44
30-39	16	41
40-49	04	10
50-59	02	05

Table 2.7 Demographic Data: Nurses		n=39
Education	n	%
Basic Nursing Education		
Diploma	12	31
Associate degree	09	23
Baccalaureate degree	17	43
Master's degree	01	03
Highest Degree Achieved		
Baccalaureate degree	27	69
Master's degree	03	08

For the home-health study, data concerning length of employment in community health nursing were not gathered. The criterion for participation in the study was a minimum of 6 months employment at the agency. None were registered nurses just entering the profession. Data collected for the ICU study showed that nursing experience working in an ICU ranged from 1 to 9 years (Table 2.8).

Table 2.8 Demographic Data: Nurses		n=19
Years of employment in ICUs	n	%
1	05	26
2	02	11
3	01	05
4	04	21
5	00	00
6	04	21
7	00	00
8	02	11
9	01	05

DATA COLLECTION METHODS

Discovering what data collection methods would be used for determining the meaning of nurse caring in the home-care setting was a challenge. Others had completed studies of caring using interviews as the sole data collection mode. In order to be faithful to the conceptual framework of symbolic interactionism, it seemed that another method would have to be devised—one in which participants could observe their own actions and interpret them to the researcher. Videotaping nurse-patient interactions and playing back the videotapes became the obvious choices.

Videotaping and playing back have contributed significantly to advances made in the study of humans, because we are best revealed in our ongoing transactions with each other. Videotaping also provides a permanent record of spontaneously interacting humans. The videotape lends itself to analysis for obtaining data (Kolb, 1978). Videotape playback provides evidence for sources of knowledge about the significance of signs and symbols that regulate and arrange communication relationships (Berger, 1978).

Videotaping was also selected because it provides participants with the opportunity to express themselves with freedom and spontaneity. As a result, responses reflected the uniqueness and individuality of each participant. Showing videotapes to the participants was found to be an effective procedure for obtaining data related to the meaning of caring in nursing. Responses to the videotape were recorded verbatim by the researcher.

As Blumer (1969) wrote:

In the observation of human conduct, one kind of item that the observer can detect readily is ... physical action ... moving an arm ... running.... Such kinds of activities can be directly perceived and easily identified; designations or descriptive accounts of them can be readily verified.... Being capable of effective validation, they do not become the cause of disputation.

However, there is another kind of item disclosed in the observation of human behavior that is of a markedly different nature, as when we observe that a person is acting aggressively, hatefully, or kindly. This kind of activity cannot be reduced to a physical act or translated into a space-time framework and still retain the character suggested by the adverbs employed. It is such a kind of act which is genuinely social; and a great many of the observations that are made of human conduct are of such acts. The observation that detects such a kind of act is different from that which reveals the physical act, and incidentally, is of a complicated nature. It is complicated in that it comes in the form of a judgment based on sensing the social relations of the situation in which the behavior occurs and on applying some social norm present in the experience of the observer; thus one observes an act as being respectful, for example, by sensing the social relation between the actor and others set by the situation, and by viewing the act from the standpoint of rights, obligations, and expectations involved in that situation.... Usually we observe the act in terms of both grasping the situation and by detecting familiar signs; ordinarily these occur together, although they do not need do so. (pp. 177-178)

HOME HEALTH STUDY

Data collection in the home health care nursing study occurred in two parts: videotaping the nurse-patient care situation and—following that—a separate interview with each participant in which the videotape was shown and answers to the research question were recorded verbatim by the researcher. For one interview, videotaping took place in the nurse's office in the agency's clinic; for the rest, videotaping occurred in the patients' homes. Data collection for the videotaping of nurse-patient situations lasted from 20 minutes to 1 hour and was conducted as quietly and unobtrusively as possible. Not all participants who were videotaped were interviewed. Several patients had been hospitalized; others had moved; still others could not be reached.

Home videocameras were relatively new technology in the early 1980s, yet the participants readily accepted the researcher and her camera. The videotape equipment was in open view and the entire episode of care was taped. Preparations for the videotaping were completed as calmly and quietly as possible to minimize any theatric or dramatic components—and in this way the situation was made as natural as possible. Often the nurses and patients would look up startled to find the researcher there, so involved were they in the nursing situation.

Data collection for the videotape playback and interviews lasted from 30 minutes to 1 hour. Interviews with the nurses took place in a quiet place in the agency; interviews with the patients took place in their homes. Occasionally, the significant other of the patient who had been present during the videotaping was present as well during the interview.

Participants were asked as they reviewed videotapes of their nurse-patient situation to:

Tell me every time that you see something in the film which indicates to you that the nurse cares about you/that you care about the client. Tell me right away and I will stop the tape to give you the time you need to describe in detail what you see.

ICU STUDY

Initially, in this second study, we made an attempt to replicate the initial data collection method of the home health study: videotaping nurse-patient care situations. Most of the ICU patients, however, were heavily sedated to enable them to tolerate respirators and other invasive, life-assisting technologies. As a result, reliable and valid informed consents were not available. Therefore, the decision was made to forego videotaping and to continue the research through separate interviews with nurses and patients about their mutual caring experiences after obtaining informed consent from all participants.

Data collection interviews with the nurses were done in quiet areas of the hospitals. Interviews with patients—or the parents in the case of neonatal and pediatric clients—who participated in the ICU study occurred after they were discharged from the hospital and were conducted either face-to-face or over the telephone. It has been found that interviewing patients concerning nurse caring while patients are still in the hospital furnishes either no information or biased information for fear that their care might be in jeopardy (P. Larson, University of California at San Francisco, personal communication, November 1983). In the ICU study, nurses and patients were asked, "How did you/How did the nurse get beyond the tubes and technology to provide caring to the patient/to you?" Responses in both studies were recorded verbatim and later transcribed.

GROUNDED THEORY

The philosophy of symbolic interactionism provides "an approach designed to yield verifiable knowledge of human group life and human conduct" (Blumer, 1969, p. 21). This method helps one to generate theory from data gathered from people living their ordinary everyday lives. It is concerned with how people make sense of problem situations in which they find themselves. Glaser and Strauss (1967) and Glaser (1978) were sources used by the researcher during data collection and analysis to guide the research for the two studies. These were the foundation for the secondary sources in nursing, such as Bowers (1988), Chenitz and Swanson (1986), Corbin (1986), Hutchinson (1986), Stern (1980), and Wilson (1989).

Grounded theory arising out of symbolic interactionism has guided these studies. Because the theory is generated from real experience, it fits "the situation being researched and works when put to use" (Glaser & Strauss, 1967, p. 3). It provides a way to deal with the amazing variability and diversity in human situations and experiences. It identifies basic (generic) social psychological and/or social structural human processes as patterns. A major concern for the grounded theorist is to determine "how contextual features of the environment influence the direction and the form of the identified social process" (Benoliel, 1996, p. 408).

Wilson (1989), following Glaser (1978), noted that in examining the data, three major types of patterns or codes were specified: substantive, selective, and theoretical. Substantive codes, also known as open codes, are words used by the participants to describe what is going on. Substantive codes include the dimensions, properties, conditions, strategies, and consequences of the problem under study. Selective coding occurs when the analyst observes similarities and differences among the substantive codes, and clusters these accordingly into related categories. The researcher also notes the range, variations, and properties of these categories. Theoretical coding begins when the analyst relates the substantive categories to one another. Glaser (1978) identified 14 families of theoretical codes (see Glaser, 1978, pp. 72-82). Prus (1996) named seven major generic social processes to be used for theoretical coding. As indicated in Glaser and Strauss (1967), other theories can be used to substantiate the grounded theory emerging from data analysis. In the instance of this monograph the theory substantiating the emerging grounded theory was that of communication theory (Watzlawick, Beavin, & Jackson, 1967).

Use of grounded theory requires the researcher to enter the research situation as personally open as possible, not deliberately bringing to it presuppositions, biases, and hypotheses. The researcher allows the situation to do the teaching—to provide the data for generating theory. While interviews were ongoing, and consistent with all grounded theory studies, the constant comparative method of data analysis was used (Glaser & Strauss, 1967). Constant comparison consists of four steps:

> Comparing incidents applicable to each category, integrating categories and their properties, delimiting the theory, and writing the theory.... Earlier stages remain in operation throughout the analysis and each provides continuous development to its successive stage until the analysis is terminated. (Glaser & Strauss, 1967, p. 105)

The interviews, which were recorded verbatim, were transcribed and read for themes that led to categories with their dimensions and properties. Theoretical sampling prompted continued interviewing until saturation was reached. As Kools, McCarthy, Durham, and Robrecht (1996) indicated:

> Once a consistent level of repetition regarding concepts and their relationships becomes evident, the analyst can assume that the collection and analysis of additional data would most probably be redundant and unproductive. At this point, theoretical saturation has been achieved. (p. 319)

The home health study was exploratory grounded theory in that at that time no previous investigation of caring in nursing had been published about caring from the perspectives of both nurses and patients–or patients' parents. The ICU study was confirmatory grounded theory as the results of the first study were verified and expanded. As stated earlier, the attempt to replicate videotaping nurse-patient care situations in the ICU was foregone as reliable and valid patient informed consents were not to be obtained. Rather, separate interviews with nurses and designated patients of those nurses were conducted to explore their mutual caring experiences.

This is one strength of the grounded-theory method of qualitative research. Grounded theory enables researchers to evaluate the data-collection situation and method, and to develop a method that is workable. Reliability and validity of the findings for the two studies were carried out with a panel of four nurse doctoral students (in the home care study), groups of nurses from the agencies in which data were collected, patients who were particularly articulate, and various audiences of nurse colleagues to whom presentations had been made.

This monograph represents the synthesis of data from the two studies. The grounded-theory method was found to be useful for secondary as well as primary analysis of the qualitative data. All the transcripts of the interviews about the videotaped playbacks of the home health care study and the transcribed interviews of the intensive care study were read and reread line by line in their entirety for the various themes of caring as components of a nurse's practice. These themes were recorded on index cards as categories. Categories and properties of categories are concepts indicated by the data and are not the data themselves. Constant comparison of category to category, category to data, and category to concept reduced these to nine concepts and their various aspects of pattern, condition, theme, dimension, property, or phase. When developing categories, the researcher noted a category once it occurred in an interview, and the several instances of that category as it occurred in the later interviews. Validation of the interpretation has been conducted with groups of nursing colleagues and people with experience with patients. The names of all nurses and patients have been changed to protect their privacy.

Chapter 3

SYNTHESIS OF
THE TWO STUDIES

Upon completion of the interviews and the constant comparative data analysis for the home health study, ever more careful scrutiny of the categories was continued. When the response categories—the properties of caring—were reviewed, it became evident that, based on postulates from communication theory (Watzlawick, Beavin, & Jackson, 1967), they could be integrated into two broad categories: responses which reflect the content of nursing, and responses which reflect the relationship between nurse and patient.

This is consistent with grounded theory methodology (Glaser & Strauss, 1967). The interview data led the researcher to discover the embedded theory through data analysis. The theory may be unique. It may also be that data are best interpreted based on the tenets of another theory. In this situation it was clear that the data represented the two irreducible categories of Watzlawick and colleagues (1967) theory of communication.

According to Watzlawick and colleagues (1967), communication consists of two irreducible aspects: content and relationship. Content includes information, while relationship constitutes the messages about the information, or metacommunication. Information or digital communication "has a highly complex and powerful logical syntax ... for the unambiguous definition of the nature of relationships" (Watzlawick et al., 1967, pp. 66-67). Relationship, metacommunication, or analogic communication "is virtually all nonverbal communication" (Watzlawick et al., 1967, p. 62). It defines the nature of the relationship and is comprised of posture, gesture, facial expression, and voice inflections (action cues); sequence, rhythm, and cadence (vocal cues); other nonverbal communications such as touch; and communication cues (objects, space) present in the context (physical setting, psychosocial setting, interpersonal relationship, history of the relationship, the culture) of the interaction (Watzlawick et al., 1967; Stuart & Sundeen, 1983).

Because the ICU study was an extension of the home-care study, for a complete understanding of the meaning of the studies to one another, the interview transcripts from both studies were analyzed together, and the findings integrated and interpreted. The synthesis is described in this chapter. Noblit and Hare (1988) contend that the synthesis of research findings is more than reviewing the literature. They "assert that ... synthesis is essentially interpretive and inductive.... [And] ... involves understanding of interpretive explanation" (p. 17). In comparing the synthesis of qualitative studies with the meta-analysis of quantitative studies, Noblit and Hare noted that meta-analysts of the positivist tradition "highlight the essentially interpretive nature of meta-analysis.... [And] point to the inductive nature of all synthesis activities" (1988, p. 15).

FINDINGS

The findings from both studies represent the universe of responses to the research questions from the studies: "Tell me every time that you see something in the film which indicates to you that the nurse cares about you/that you care about the client" and "How did you/How did the nurse get beyond the tubes and technology to provide caring to the patient/to you?"

Nine categories emerged from the constant comparison method of data analysis of the interviews of the two studies. The content aspect of the communication of caring in nursing was revealed in four categories: physical care, health promotion, health assessment, and patient advocacy. The relationship aspect was revealed in five categories: dialogue; conveying progress and hope; attachment; knowing patients, families, and significant others; and concern.

One's knowledge about relationship is learned by development of bodily senses and by development of personal skills through encounters with other humans. It becomes tacit knowledge. One's knowledge about nursing content is learned through academic studies and then made one's own through practicing in nursing situations. It too becomes tacit knowledge (Polanyi & Prosch, 1975). Together, knowledge of relationship and nursing content of the communication of nurse caring brings humanity into that practice–a combination that is a powerful tool toward human well-being. Here lies the explanation of how the content and relationship aspects of the communication of caring in nursing become irreducible; they are brought together through tacit knowing.

Other topics which emerged were balance, differentiating between caring and nursing, ethical concerns, examples of caring and not caring, stages of caring, structural caring, and time. These topics will be discussed following the presentation of participants' responses. All contribute to understanding the theory of the communication of caring in nursing.

Some categories that were present in the original studies do not appear in the synthesis. This is the result of reading the interviews anew as a whole in preparation for synthesis and interpretation. As in the home care and ICU studies, the basic social process continued to be identified as the communication of caring in nursing and the two aspects of communication—content and relationship. Participant response categories reflecting content are presented first in the following discussion.

PARTICIPANT RESPONSES

In the home-care study, patients' response categories were drawn from responses to the videotape playback by 20 patients. Nineteen categories were identified: 15 reflected content, and 4, relationship. In the ICU study patients' response categories were drawn from interviews with 12 patients. Nineteen categories were also identified from the patients' responses: 5 categories reflected content and 14 reflected relationship.

Nurse response categories in the home-care study were drawn from the interviews following the videotape playbacks with 20 nurses. From the total of 19 categories, nurses contributed to 15: 8 were related to content, 7 to relationship. Nurse response categories in the ICU study were drawn from interviews with 19 nurses. Nurses contributed data to 7 content categories, and 19 relationship categories. Nine dimensions comprise the theory of the communication of caring in nursing. In the presentation that follows, participant response categories have been synthesized; there is no separation of nurse from patient responses.

PARTICIPANT RESPONSE CATEGORIES: CONTENT

These categories were derived from the synthesis of the interviews from the home-care and ICU studies. Four major categories were identified that relate to the content, information, or technology of nursing: physical care, health promotion, health assessment, and patient advocacy. Some interviews had several instances in the category. Some categories also had several properties, which were explicated in the discussion of the category.

Physical Care

Physical care is an obvious caring activity of nursing. It included the dimensions of physical care itself, comfort, being gentle and careful while protecting, physical limitations, and positioning.

Physical care. Physical care involved changing diapers and dressings, giving baths and shampoos, treating wounds, and burping babies. It meant that when nurses were providing care to unconscious patients, "I would tell them first what I'm going to do, stroke first, comfort before I do something, and do comfort measures after." Another nurse caring for an unconscious patient said the following:

I did a lot of caring for him as a patient. One way was physical care. He was ventilated, had intravenous feedings, narcotics for pain, and the Pavulon. When I think of caring for him, I'd think of the things he couldn't do, such as talking.

I'd tell what I [was going to do] before touching him. He had a fear of suffocation, so I'd tell him what I would do. I'd help him breathe. Before suctioning him, I'd put Vaseline to his lips. I bathed him ... [shaved him and gave] passive range of motion ... I'd respond to him as a responder.

Being gentle and careful. A nurse "uses skin prep to protect the fragile skin from daily dressing changes." The patient in this interview also commented on the nurse's precautionary actions as viewed on the videotape:

She's protecting my bed. She's careful in her technique and in not hurting me.... She's careful where she puts the dressing, not close to open areas. And she's careful when she takes off the bandage that she doesn't tear the skin.

Another patient noted that "she [the nurse] uses Maalox to protect the skin from the tape."

Comfort. The comfort dimension included the nursing content aspect of communication through the actions of "placing a pad in the wheelchair for comfort," and "placing the bandage so he's comfortable." It also showed that comfort had a relationship aspect of communication through statements such as, "trying to lessen her pain by taking her mind off it," and "We [the parents] felt the staff were very comforting [to us]." This is an example of the irreducible nature of the two aspects of communication, content, and relationship.

Physical limitations. Physical limitations as a dimension of physical care were taken into account by "opening and closing the client's buttons, thus recognizing her inability;" "taking into account his hearing loss;" "being realistic about [the limitation]."

Positioning. Positioning is addressed in the comfort dimension. It also meant wrapping a dressing securely; preserving modesty; "using the kind of dressing the patient wanted, how he wanted it."

Health Promotion

This nursing content category implicitly included health teaching. Nurses validated patients' information about diets: "She is teaching me to cut down on salt, and teaching me about the salt." And the nurse in the same interview said, "I am helping him to be independent in his diet."

Nurses taught about medications and about social services (e.g., Medicaid). They taught patients about the diseases and other health problems and how to manage these diseases and problems. They corrected misconceptions and myths. A comment from a patient follows: "One nurse developed a great deal of knowledge on the subject [heart attack]. She encouraged me to ask questions. Just talking about it and getting the terminology helped. I was in the ICU 10 days."

Nurses taught about the healing process of wounds. They taught and explained "what's going on with a piece of equipment."

Neonatal intensive care unit nurses taught parents of infants in the neonatal nursery how to become involved with the care of their baby:

I teach them how to do safflower oil rubs. I encourage them to bring in tapes of parents' voices [to use] following procedures to associate [with] something positive, tapes of voices or music played at home, a tape of love sounds, fetal heart beat, placenta swish with music. I encourage them to bring home a blanket for the baby's smell.

A mother's response was:

I didn't know I could do things like changing the diaper, taking the temp, assisting with some of the techniques.... She was very patient. She taught me to hold Elaine. She taught me how to use the machines if I came in.... She taught me to understand what would send off the alarm. She taught me to identify what a problem was, and what was not. She taught me about the oxygen [after Elaine was discharged], ... at the clinic they suggested some meds that Elaine had already been on and taken off. When I got back I called the primary and told her. She didn't say anything against, but she helped me understand what the meds were for and why. She helped me understand the use of the meds—Lasix and Theophyllin for irregular heart beat.... They thought the Theophyllin was necessary. But the dose was too strong and Elaine was not sleeping. The primary helped me to understand why she was not sleeping. Then I was able to call the pediatrician here, who called to lower the dose. Now it's not affecting her.

Nurses taught mothers about immunizations, the growth and development of their children and themselves, safety, and their own need for rest and diversion. Nurses also taught members of the extended family: "The teaching she did for me, she did for my husband and sister-in-law, too."

Nurses synthesized knowledge they had about the client with knowledge about health in order to teach appropriately: "I am fitting the client's information about her role as mother as a teacher of children to start good eating habits and linking themes about cholesterol, salt, sugar to reinforce that role."

Thus, the nurse's teaching reinforces the patient's behavior changes. The patient in this interview recognized the nurse's teaching ability:

She doesn't try to tell you. She gives suggestions. She knows that losing weight is not an easy thing. She gives you ideas you can live with, [that are] not stringent.... She gives good helpful suggestions.... She doesn't stress diet, but changing your way of thinking, substituting and keeping yourself busy ... behavior modification is more important than thinking diet. She stresses that health is important, not being thin and starving yourself to be thin.

Neonatal intensive care unit nurses say they:

[E]xplain simply [to parents] the tubes, IV, monitor, the dots on the baby. We encourage [the parents] to touch [and talk to] them as they've been "hearing your voice" for 9 months.... We explain the O_2 concentration with ways to look for improvement for the baby.

Neonatal intensive care unit nurses also taught mothers how to provide breast milk to their babies:

My baby weighed 1 lb. 5 oz. at birth. The nurses helped me to use a breast pump and start breast feeding in the hospital. One nurse had also breast fed and she was able to help me. Essentially I pumped for 5 months. The nurses supported me a great deal.

Elaine's mother said: "After Elaine was strong enough to be out of the incubator for short times, she helped me to nurse. She encouraged me to keep on. By the time we got Elaine home, she'd never had a bottle of formula."

A second nurse asked a mother to demonstrate to her the exercises for her child "for the evaluation of safe practice."

Health teaching. An integral part of the nursing role was health teaching. It was critical to patients' well being and healing. What the nurses were doing in these interviews was not just health teaching, the content aspect of the communication of nurse caring: They were simultaneously communicating the relationship aspects of caring through patience, reassurance, and support.

Health Assessment

Health assessment also included the dimensions of health and physical assessment, examining, and observing. It involved the usual nursing actions of monitoring blood pressures, temperatures, and pulses; checking the machines; listening to lungs and heart sounds; assessing and measuring limbs; assessing activities of daily living including sleeplessness and nocturnal voiding, pain and discomfort, hallucinations, X-ray and lab results, diet and fluid intake, and details of support systems.

In ICU settings, health assessment was also involved. A neonatal ICU nurse expressed it this way: "You really are concerned with vital signs and stabilizing ... getting to know what's normal for the baby and what he gets stressed out on; you look for the baby's time out signals, that is, mottling, apnea."

A second nurse concurred:

I think in the beginning it's hard to get beyond the tubes. On the first day or so, you're concentrating on keeping the baby alive. Then you pick up on cues of what keeps the baby happy, when he's ready or not by his activity, monitor info, color, facial expression such as grimacing.

Health assessment also meant, "I ensure he has meds enough so as not to run out." It meant "making sure everything is okay," "checking," observing through "continual assessment through the bath." And for a patient who had a tracheostomy tube in place, "I had to observe her nonverbal behavior to figure out what was going on with her. I knew the minute I walked in the door what kind of day she was having by the expression on her face."

Health assessment also incorporated the category Prevention. A nurse working with a young mother with 9-month-old developmentally delayed twin daughters warned the mother about the babies' hoop earrings because the babies were playing with each other and tugging at the earrings.

Patient Advocacy

Another category in the content aspect of the communication of caring in nursing was that of patient advocacy. It consisted of four dimensions: being a patient advocate, following through or following up, providing resources, and going above and beyond.

Nurses both advocated (verb) for and were advocates (noun) for patients and their families. According to Merriam-Webster's Collegiate Dictionary (1995), an "advocate (noun) is one that pleads the cause of another; one that defends or maintains a cause or proposal; advocate (verb) is to plead in favor of, to support." This linguistic information caused the writer to review relationship categories of the communication of caring in nursing—namely, dimensions of conveying progress and hope: encouraging, reassuring, and supporting. Here is a category whose meaning demonstrates the irreducible nature of communication. Content and relationship aspects can be separated, but only artificially.

Being a patient advocate. A patient described how his nurse was an advocate for him: "She keeps in touch with [my practitioner] to find out what's to be done. She gets through right away. They give us the runaround and get back 5 days later.... She has been instrumental in getting the tube changed."

An ICU nurse related how she advocated special care for a special "pedi case" on the adult ICU:

> She came here [because] they wanted to Swan her, and there's not too many on the pedi ICU. She has Rubenstein's taboid syndrome: mental retardation with some problems with the growth hormones.... She's 17, a pretty special kid.... I'm always watching the physicians, too. As when they're ordering something, I may not agree—I'm watching out for her best interests and the family, too. I say, "Can't you do it this way?" I have them do better than they routinely do [because] she's handled by both pediatricians and surgeons. The surgeons think of her as an adult; I try to keep the pedi in the perspective with them. These physicians are not in much contact with children. They mainly deal with adults.

Another ICU nurse first talked about how she learned to see the baby beyond the tubes, and then discussed being a patient advocate:

Now I go out of my way to be a patient advocate. Last night the docs wanted to do an arterial stick. I went out of my way to assure it was really needed. It seems that many of them do not think about [the baby]. They say, "I have to get the blood."

A third nurse considered how she had become a patient advocate for a baby in the neonatal ICU:

My first primary had chest tubes, intravenous feedings, central lines. We had to do chest compressions. I focused on the parents and their needs ... it was taking care of the whole family. They were Jehovah Witnesses and I had to be very, very sensitive in talking to them, especially to the father. I used his feelings to care for the baby as having similar feelings as the father. I was sensitive about the invasive procedures as I became the advocate for the baby as their rights were taken away. The parents are your major source to bring you down to the baby. It's not just taking care of the tubes.... The medical staff didn't feel that the baby should die ... so we went to court....

I have a very different position. I let the parents know that I was in a neutral position. I would be an advocate against aggressive treatment. I would respect their rights.

In the previous discussion about health promotion and teaching, the mother talked about how her daughter's primary nurse taught her about her daughter's Theophyllin. This incident also unveiled the nurse's patient advocacy role as well. The nurse helped the mother understand how to present the situation to her pediatrician, who called the consulting physician in a distant city, who then rectified the situation.

Following through or following up. Following through or following up was a dimension of patient advocacy in communicating caring in nursing. In two instances, nurses followed through with their patient to ensure the patient's needs were understood. "I cared for her for two days on the step-down unit and established a good rapport with the other nurses. When I was back in the ICU, I continued to visit the patient on the step down unit." In the second incident, the child's mother said, "I liked Lisa, my primary care nurse, a lot. One day [my child] had a setback and they tried to call me, but I wasn't home yet. Lisa called me from her home [to let me know]."

In these ways nurses were champions for their patients. They promoted situations that enhanced patients' and families' well-being. From the patients' point of view, they defended the patient from unnecessary medical care.

Resources. The dimension of patient advocacy called resources represented the activities of identifying, obtaining, referring, supplying, and using. The need for resources occurred as a result of assessing a patient's or a family's health, and of providing physical care.

Nurses referred patients to Meals-on-Wheels, homemaker services, home health aides, day care, speech evaluation, and to the source for food stamps. They obtained and supplied equipment such as a Hoyer Lift, surgical dressings, and other materials. Elaine's mother recalled: "She was so small, there were no clothes to fit. Another mother had left tiny baby pajamas and one put them on Elaine. My nurse made a dress for Elaine for Christmas."

Nurses ascertained if parents had transportation to keep appointments and made arrangements to supply it if they did not. Patients and nurses viewed these activities within the purview of caring in nursing.

Going above and beyond. A dimension of patient advocacy which was also closely linked with the relationship category of conveying progress and hope was going above and beyond. An example was Elaine's mother's statement: "She went beyond the call of duty. She let us know what the baby was doing. She'd fill me in on the extras. She helped me to nurse; she'd call when they were ready to feed." Elaine's mother also recalled an incident about breast feeding. "Once she had formula. A nurse had gone and given it. My nurse was so angry. 'This mom's supplying milk for the baby. Let's give it to the baby.' She took the initiative to make sure others used it."

PARTICIPANT RESPONSE CATEGORIES: RELATIONSHIP

Five major categories were uncovered in the synthesis that described the relationship aspects of the communication of caring in nursing: dialogue; conveying progress and hope; attachment; knowing patients, families, significant others; and concern. Relationship aspects characterize the meaning, message, metacommunication, and expression about the content—the information aspect of communication.

The Dialogue

Dialogue—feeling caring through speech—that occurs among the nurse, patient, and the patient's significant other was identified as a significant relationship aspect of the communication of caring. Two main categories were (a) verbal communication and (b) nonverbal communication. Each of these major categories had several dimensions that are described below.

Verbal communication. This relationship category demonstrated nurse caring through the usual actions that people associate with ordinary, everyday communication. This category has many dimensions including: talking, telling what was found, listening, humor and laughing together, clarifying, asking questions, telling what is going to be done, talking about feelings, and explaining.

Talking. Talking meant "to let [the patient] talk without interrupting." It meant "communicating with [the patient]." "Interacting." "General conversation." Talking to meant caring to a mother who, while reviewing the videotape of her baby, the nurse, and herself, commented: "I like the way she talks to him and smiles at him. She's holding him just at the right distance for him to see her." This mother went on to say,

What [the nurse] did was what all the nurses did ... they're accustomed to taking care of babies. There were some nurses who'd hold, hug, and kiss them—they're the nurses who show they care about the babies. I never considered him being in an intensive care nursery. He was just in a nursery and needed to be taken care of. I never saw it as technical.

Several nurses and mothers of babies in the neonatal intensive care units and pediatric ICUs indicated that "talking to babies was part of caring." "Holding, cuddling, and talking" were words that occurred together in several interviews. It was by talking to parents that "you get to know what the family is feeling about the hospitalization." One nurse said the following about her relationship with an adult patient:

Because the patient had a trach, I had to ... explain ... things to her. For her that would mean a lot. She needed a lot of explanation. It meant translating and helping her to communicate with other health care workers ... reiterating for clearer communication.

For other nurses, it meant "explaining what I was about to do," or "explaining events to him while correcting misconceptions."

Telling what was found. In talking to patients, nurses "tell what she finds," and "tell what's going on," thus providing important information to patients or their families. One patient said, "She's telling me about the foot [because] I'm worried about the infection." "She tells me about my BP." Many nurses working in ICUs telephone family members to let them know "if it's a positive new event. We call them as well [if it is not], even if the docs are to call. [We call] first as the nurse is the one who sees them and knows them."

Listening. Listening is an important aspect of relationship. Patients noted that their nurse "listened intently," "listens good," "listens to personal problems ... personal concerns." One patient stated, "She's a good listener. It's okay to tell her how I feel." "She follows my directions ... in caring for my foot."

A nurse said:

I'm listening while I'm doing the dressing. I'm able to filter out and identify what is important.... In listening to her, I'm supportive of other nurses, while letting her know her comments are important.... We discuss world events or soap opera events. I participate through listening.... Talking with her is communicating, listening, responding to events of care with the new home health aide. Communication is very important between patient and nurse ... I listen to complaints and respond, respond to the changes in symptoms she experiences with multiple sclerosis.

This nurse also indicated that "communicating with the husband [helps him] to feel [he is] an important part of what's going on." Other nurses report they "listen to the family talk about concerns."

Humor and laughing together. There were several incidents of humor and laughing together. Almost all the reported incidents occurred in home care settings, undoubtedly indicating the caring relationship these nurses and patients were able to establish over the course of many home visits (seven or more). Sometimes the humor was associated with a patient's habit: "humor about her cigarette addiction." At other times, the laughter and humor may have arisen because of anxiety and discomfort generated in the situation.

Here is a nurse's comment about the videotape showing her interaction with a patient: "I am returning to the original complaint of tingling, reviewing and trying to identify a possible cause. I am reviewing the parameters of the disease obliquely. I am touching her. Now there is laughter, a sense of humor."

Nurses used laughter and humor to help patients to relax. A patient expressed his appreciation that the ICU nurses "tried within the time pressure to laugh at my jokes and my attempts to be normal."

Nurses and patients laughing together demonstrated "enjoying the patient's statements. It demonstrates that I enjoy the visit with the patient as a person."

In one nursing situation, both the nurse and patient commented on the lack of humor:

NURSE: This is an uncharacteristic interaction in that it's so quiet; his wife is not sitting on the bed. We always ask personal questions, tease. The [presence of] the camera changed the interaction.

PATIENT: We're usually not so quiet. We wanted everything to be good, not fooling around, teasing.

Clarifying. Nurses in these studies clarified feelings and discomforts as well as how a resource was to be used: "I'm clarifying it's a supplement, not to be substituted for a meal."

Asking questions. Patients commented that when the nurse asks questions, "She is inquisitive. She inquires about things." "Her questions are not intrusive. They're sympathetic."

Telling what is going to be done. Nurses also tell what is going to be done when providing physical care to both conscious and unconscious patients. In regard to unconscious patients, nurses stated, "I tell them first what I'm going to do. I stroke first, and [provide] comfort before I do something, then do comfort measures after." "I'd tell him what I do before touching him." A nurse in the home-care study described working with a patient by saying, "I attempt to calm her by explaining the activities as I do them."

Talking about feelings. Two nurses described talking to patients about their feelings: One said, "I am listening closely, verbalizing, acknowledging the patient's feelings." "I am listening and then talking about the client's feelings."

Explaining. Another nurse helped a patient with a tracheostomy communicate by:

> [E]xplaining things to her—for her—that would mean a lot; she needed a lot of explanation, translating, helping her to communicate with other health care workers ... I am reiterating for clearer communication, taking time to understand her ... not being in a rush to go anywhere.

Nonverbal Communication. Nonverbal communication has several dimensions such as touching, eye contact, holding, playing with babies, and other nonverbal communication.

Touching. Several nurses mentioned that there were "ways of touching" that conveyed caring. "I touch even when I don't need to. She's conscious of the touch." "I show caring concern via interest in her foot, touching, hands on. The foot is the focus of this relationship!" "I use touching as part of physical assessment when evaluating the lungs. The client likes the touching." "While doing physical care, it's not ordinarily necessary to massage ... the touch is important to her."

An ICU nurse used the example of hair washing as caring. The following is from comments about her videotape:

> I'm supporting her getting up. I'm changing her position, helping her to be comfortable. I'm explaining what I'm about to do. I'm looking at her, making eye contact when answering questions. I'm allowing her to make decisions and asking her opinion. We're switching her to another chair; checking the temperature of the shampoo water. I'm asking her how she's doing several times. Now I'm drying her hair with a towel. All through there is gentle touching.... Hair washing shows that you care. I always do it on my unit, but many of the nurses don't. But I just think it makes the patients feel so much better.

The nurse working with the patient who had a tracheostomy used "gentle touch" to get her patient's attention. And the ICU nurse working with the 17-year-old with Rubenstein's taboid syndrome said she: "communicated with her by watching her.... When I turn her, I stroke her ... I do this gently [because] this is a pedi patient, as compared to an adult: the tubes are pedi tubes, my touch is lighter."

Many nurses working with babies and children, whether in neonatal ICUs, pediatric ICUs, or at home, spoke about stroking, holding, cuddling, rocking, and playing with them and identified these actions as caring.

Parents commented on nurses playing with the babies, "not ignoring them." It is particularly clear in the subcategory about touch how irreducible the content and relationship aspects of touch are. By touching during health assessment, bathing, and physical care nurses conveyed support, human-to-human contact, and concern.

Eye contact. Both nurses and patients mentioned eye contact. In one interview, the nurse's first comment on viewing the videotape was about "the amount of eye contact present." A second nurse who had been working with a baby and was viewing a videotape of the experience, exclaimed, "Eye-to-eye contact. See! She's looking at me!" The nurse working with the patient with a tracheostomy said this when observing the videotape, "Eye contact, being face-to-face." Another neonatal ICU nurse talked about a baby: "When I was on vacation and I returned, he looked me over, up and down. By the end of the day, I felt he'd accepted me and knew me. He'll check you out if he doesn't know you."

Holding. Both nurses and parents discussed holding, cuddling, and rocking babies as indicative of caring. One mother while looking at the videotape said, "She's holding him just at the right distance for him to see her." Two patients also considered "the nurse's holding her hand" as caring.

Playing with babies. Parents and nurses regarded playing with babies as representing caring by nurses. On viewing the videotape one mother stated, "[The nurse] recognizes that Alice wanted her attention, and she picked her up rather than ignoring her." Another young mother said, "She shows caring when she's touching him. When she fixes his hat, you know she cares if he's comfortable when she's playing with him."

Other nonverbal communication. The sound qualities of the nurse's voice drew comments in several interviews in each study. "My voice is low and soothing. My approach is quiet and non-threatening." "I sound enthusiastic." Patients commented on "politeness," "warmth and sensitivity," "a quiet manner and voice." One elderly man said, "The way she tells me to breathe when listening to my heart, let's me know how I am." One patient mentioned that the nurse's smiling indicated she cared for her.

Conveying Progress and Hope

The relationship category called Conveying Progress and Hope had many dimensions including: concentrating, building self-esteem, empathizing, comforting, reassuring, encouraging, fostering autonomy, involving patients and significant others, preparing, supporting, understanding, being equal, accommodating, being available, demonstrating competence, being willing to answer questions, respecting, referring to a patient by name, being considerate, expressing compassion, and trusting.

Concentrating. Concentrating had eight aspects: taking time, doing extra, going above and beyond, being interested, doing normal things, focusing, practicing patience, and doing little things.

Concentrating for these nurses and patients meant paying attention over long periods. A nurse in a pediatric ICU said:

> You overlook the tubes as you're so used to them. You deal with the baby as a baby, yet knowing that possibly he'll get into trouble. You get to know the kids by taking care of them for ... long periods of time, at least a month. You're interacting with them a lot. You care for no more than three children in here. It's concentrated care.

A patient's significant other stated, "I feel as if there's a healing process in this kind of personal attention." And a nurse said the following as she viewed the videotape:

> This is continuous caring: I know how I am; I was not sure how I came across ... it's intense; she has my undivided attention as I assist her. Here [I am] watching, undistracted by the camera, total involvement.

The subcategory, taking time, was reported by nurses and patients or parents. Patients noted that "[the nurse] takes time to talk." One parent commented, "If they had time, they would do things like play, rock, and talk to the babies." This same baby's nurse stated that "it is important to find time to hold, sit, talk, touch, and cuddle babies." Patients also noticed that the nurse "doesn't waste time."

One nurse found that "to understand [a patient and not be] in a rush helps. I am giving her time, but keeping time limits." Nurses "take time to talk of incidentals," "to do social amenities," "to do extra." They also noticed that they spend "more extra time when they were attached to a baby."

More patients than nurses commented about nurses "doing extra." One nurse for a very old patient said, "I am doing extra for him ... I come before work to put in his eye drops without charge ... I am concerned about how he is making payments for his meds." And the patient said, "She's a very nice nurse who goes above and beyond ... she does extra, she always left enough supplies."

Examples of ways nurses "go above and beyond" in providing care to their patients were described by patients as follows. "She has stopped when she was not supposed to, just to check up.... She stopped by to teach me the use of the new BP cuff." "Sometimes she goes above and beyond by correcting the defective equipment."

Being interested was described as "interested in their patients" and "tried to include [the patient] in everything." They "shared stories [and] events in their personal lives." One nurse cogently stated:

I'm interested in the hospitalization, in the events of the hospitalization, in what happened. I'm interested in how she's doing, how she's
feeling now. I'm taking an interest in her family. I'm interested in the
problems associated with the chemotherapy.

Nurses also revealed "being interested in what she has to say," and
"I'm interested in this lady."

Doing normal things, an additional dimension, was considered by
nurses to include talking to, feeding, hair washing, and bathing "while
always watching for changes" as indicative of caring. Sometimes doing
normal things meant "normalizing the intensive care situation":

> When I walk in with the unconscious gravely ill child, I find out from
> the parents what the kid looks like ... I clean them up, take off extra
> electrodes, [and] straighten up the bed. I have a child look like a child.
> If there's emphasis on the tubes, I clean up the bloody nasogastric
> tubes and clean up the kid's face from saliva.... I put on a gown. If
> they're really white, I'll cover the pillow with a colored case. I advo-
> cate cutting down on some of the machines. Get rid of the moni-
> tors—that's one less piece of equipment [for] the parents to deal with.
> I care for these kids. I find activity that's appropriate—I'm not big on
> [turning on] the video—toys, music for the babies, toddlers, especially
> for unconscious kids.

Focusing, another dimension, means to "remain patient-centered in
caring." It also means to "redirect the interview."

Patience was exhibited when concentrating on patients and their care.
A sample comment was, "She has the patience of an angel."

In the incident with Elaine's mother discussed earlier under Health
Promotion, the nurse demonstrated patience. She also demonstrated concentrating, in her ability to focus on the child's needs. Concentrating also
is evident in the length of the relationship this family had with the nurse.
She continued to act as their primary nurse even though the baby had
been discharged from the hospital, an example of "going above and beyond" as well.

One nurse talked about how "doing little things" demonstrated caring:

> I provide the little things, a favorite TV show, a book, music; that's
> where the family comes in ... washing hair, doing things for him,
> setting the cards up, reading them to him ... the little things: the
> extra blanket, the extra exercise. I take time to do things more fre-
> quently if they're going to help the person.

Building self-esteem. Building self-esteem is an important aspect of
patients' return to health. Patients commented that the nurse was "a mo-
rale builder." Some nurses remarked that they were "reinforcing [patients']
getting well process." Another nurse said, "I respond to her talking; I
don't ignore it."

One patient noted the nurse's "appreciation of an individual's capability to decide ... [saying] I am reluctant to cut the aide, she eases me into a responsible decision." That patient's minister also commented on the nurse's behavior by saying, "Rather than this is the way it is and tough!, she involves you in owning that decision to figure out how many hours [you'll need the aide].... This demonstrates a healing respect for the self."

Empathizing. This dimension was revealed through the following statement by several nurses: "I really relate to her pain." It was also seen when nurses talked of being close, and being there. One patient said, "She says what I think. I feel her concern that these are her troubles."

The nurse in this nursing situation explained her actions seen on the videotape, "I moved in, physically closer." Another nurse commented, "I identify with, I feel empathy with the mother's hectic schedule about the problems with [the child]." And a third nurse, in commenting on her videotape, said, "I am sitting with her; my body position is close to the patient ... I allow the patient to touch me."

Another nurse said, "I am touching her arm, getting physically closer ... you don't even have to say anything anymore—you can just read her, empathizing with what she's going through."

A patient provided this long explanation of the importance of being there:

> In the situation in the heart attack, everyone has a function, a medical function. Yet I think for myself the event went through my mind, and unless I maintained contact and verbal communication, I had the option to choose to die or to live. Dying was not offensive or scary. It was not a clear-cut decision. If I had gotten coldhearted treatment, or uncaring treatment, or a lack of response, I might have decided otherwise.

Comforting. The concept comforting in response to patients' or parents' distress appeared in the dimensions of being gentle and careful, and positioning in the content category Physical Care. The consolation aspect of comfort is demonstrated in the comment, "I am trying to lessen the pain by taking her mind off it through diversion," said one nurse while viewing the videotape. A parent found "the staff were very comforting."

Reassuring. Reassuring was an additional dimension of conveying progress and hope. One nurse commented:

> I am reinforcing the healing. I give positive reinforcement for both the patient and the caretaker, leading to his increased security [about] her caring for him. I give positive reinforcement about the healing and about her dressing technique. I am reassuring them.

The patient in this nursing situation remarked, "She gives pep talks." Another patient stated, "She uplifts the attitude toward the sick." Patients' comments were "She is reassuring me that I'm doing a good job." "She's reassuring about the foot ulcer. I'm hoping it will heal soon."

Encouraging. Encouraging patients is also an aspect of conveying progress and hope. Some quotes from nurses include the following. "I am showing her that exercises *are* strengthening her limbs." "I am encouraging her about the blood pressure." "I am encouraging her to do better and more." "I give positive encouragement to the caretaker as well." A patient noted that the nurse's comments about her foot healing encouraged her. Another nurse stated:

> I am giving her a feeling of progress by confirming her steadiness. [When] I compliment her to reinforce her weight gain ... I also am reminding her where she was and how far she has come. I am reminding her of her progress. I give positive reinforcement about the progress. I compliment her positive attitude.

Fostering autonomy. In the dimension of fostering autonomy, nurses talked about "getting her to be independent," or "allowing her to be in an autonomous role, and yet I am concerned about her independence and autonomy." Health teaching also fosters autonomy.

Involving patients, families, and significant others. Involving patients and significant others in the patient's care sometimes meant to "respond to her requests." At other times, it meant to "communicate with the husband to [have him] feel an important part of what's going on." One patient characterized it as, "The teaching she did for me, my husband, and sister-in-law." A parent stated, "The nurse began teaching them from the first time [we] entered the unit until the baby was discharged."

Several nurses revealed actions similar to the following, "If I'm giving care, I give them the opportunity to do it. I ask them to bring things, clothes—families do make it homey. They bring the holidays in."

Preparing. The dimension, preparing, had two meanings: One had to do with future goals, and the other had to do with anticipating immediate discomforts. Nurses working with patients "identified a goal," "seek mutual goals, negotiate." In situations requiring physical care nurses "anticipate making her [the patient] comfortable via suggestions," and "anticipate certain discomforts she will encounter."

Supporting. Nurses working with patients in ICUs and community settings provide support to patients and parents. "I'm supporting her feeling of progress." "I'm confirming ... her medications." One nurse commented on the patient's behavior on the videotape: "She seems to react positively to guidance and caring. She seeks direction as well."

Understanding. Demonstrating understanding is another means to communicate progress and hope to patients. "I am showing understanding about how she needs to be part of the family even when dieting," a nurse said. And the patient in this interview commented, "She doesn't try to tell you, she is understanding." And another patient concerning another nurse said, "She is sensible and understanding." A mother of a baby in a neonatal ICU indicated, "It's hard to say specifically what is caring. It's in their manner ... the cuddling, loving, and understanding."

Being equal. Being equal also conveys progress and hope. A nurse expressed this while viewing the videotape when she stated, "The client is educating the nurse when the nurse doesn't know the answer, and that's OK." Another nurse noted on viewing the videotape, "We are sitting close at the same level." A patient said that the nurses "care about all their patients equally."

Accommodating. Nurses' accommodation of patients' requests and expectations also convey progress and hope. One said, "We accommodate our schedules mutually." The patient in this situation said, "She visits at my convenience." A nurse working in a pediatric ICU remarked, "You make accommodations for the quads at home to visit."

Availability. The nurses also were available to patients: "I am identifying that I will return and exactly when." "I am setting up the appointment to instruct the new homemaker." "I am making sure that she had the nurse's phone number in case of a problem." A patient in the homecare study commented, "She comes when I need her," and went on to discuss an instance of overdose of insulin. And "she lets me know that she's available, 'If you need me, call.' [She encourages me] to call her for any changes."

Competence. The nurse's competence also conveyed progress and hope to patients. One patient said, "She is thorough ... she examines the foot closely ... takes the pulse, measures the foot for change, teaching me how to care for the foot." A second patient stated simply, "You couldn't get better advice off doctors."

A patient from a cardiac ICU commented on nurses' competence:

It was in a sense their professionalism. I was impressed by ... how hard they worked.... I was impressed by them and their knowledge ... they would take time to answer questions and make available the information they impart about illness, the information they pass on. Nurses are more important than the doctors. They used more a layman's way of presenting information. They know the types of questions and the responses people ask.... I think I'm impressed by technology. I do computer programming. I'm a gadget person. Yet, ... I was so impressed by the efforts put in by the whole staff.

Willing to answer questions. Nurses' willingness to answer questions also conveyed progress and hope. A patient stated, "She's explaining the healing process.... She's always willing to answer questions." When completing a patient's health assessment, the nurse commented about the activities on the videotape, "I am identifying her problems and addressing her complaint."

Respecting. Communicating respect to a patient also contributes to progress and hope. One patient stated, "[The nurse] involves you in owning that decision to figure out ... your abilities rather than imposing the decision. This shows respect, a healing respect for the self."

Referring to a patient by name. Besides conveying respect this also contributed to conveying progress and hope. Nurses and patients or parents commented on this. Two nurses working in a neonatal ICU said, "Each of them has a nickname." A mother remarked, "She shows caring when she says his name."

Considerate. The concept being considerate occurred when a patient indicated, "She visits at my convenience, she is considerate." A second patient noted, "She is inquisitive with concern; she shows thoughtfulness ... and consideration."

Compassionate. The concept of being compassionate is another aspect of conveying progress and hope. One ICU patient stated, "She is sympathetic and shows compassion." A mother of a baby in a neonatal ICU said, "The nurses were compassionate when doing blood gasses because [the patients] were uncomfortable."

Trusting. Trust was identified when a nurse commented, "I'm telling the patient to trust the information she gives me. I don't have to see everything she can do." The patient stated, "She communicates that if she is not aware of something, I feel free to tell her what I think."

ATTACHMENT

Attachment was identified in many interviews with patients and nurses. Of these congruence was present between five nurse-patient pairs. Attachment indicates mutuality in these relationships.

NURSE: I am enjoying her. There is mutual enjoyment of the visit.

PATIENT: I look forward to her coming. She makes you feel as if she cares for you alone.

In a second nurse-patient pair, the nurse stated, "This is more than a nurse-patient relationship. The patient is as interested in me personally as I am in her. We exchange stories." And the patient simply says, "She enjoys my company."

A third nurse-patient pair said the following:

PATIENT: We are sharing information about our families.

NURSE: Thank you for letting me look at the tape ... I ... see how much he's lost in the last month, and since I know I'm leaving in a month, I wonder how much time we have left together. [Cried.] I knew termination was going to be hard, but seeing it here on the tape, it really confronts me head on.

A fourth nurse-patient pair and the patient's minister upon viewing the videotape also agreed about the attachment:

NURSE: I demonstrate that I enjoy the visit with the patient as a person.

PATIENT: It's a similar feeling to a young daughter, the feeling bounces on me and bounces back again. It's a close relationship; the same feeling of family and friendship, the same feeling as Christmas, a warm feeling of friendship.

PATIENT'S MINISTER: What impresses me [is] the personal level she relates: She knows you, and her knowledge of you is similar to a daughter.

One patient said, "I could listen to her 24 hours a day." Another patient said, "It's like your own. It feels like I'm her own mother, she's like a daughter. I care for her. I can tell her things like she was one of my own." And a nurse said, "I've come to love this couple."

Nurses in intensive care settings also discussed attachment. One nurse commented:

Through my attachment, I let others know how to take care of him. This is what you do.... They get new primaries and you let them know what the baby is like. You get very attached, possessive. You help them to grow.... She had a terrible time eating, yet you have to let them grow, too, like holding her own bottle. Attachment influences care. The more attached you are, the more extra time you spend with them. I push harder, knowing their limits [but I'm] patient when they're having a hard day.

When a baby is not doing well, and you're attached, it's harder to relay info other than good news. You cry, but not necessarily here.

Another nurse commented, "No one else wanted to take care of her because she was so demanding, but I became attached to her."

Knowing patients, families, significant others

Family members, nurses, and patients agreed that having knowledge about patients and families contributed to the kind of care the nurse provided. Taking care of patients over long periods provided nurses with information about them. One nurse said, "I know the minute I walked in the door what kind of day she was having by the expression on her face, and she knew me well, too."

A baby's mother stated, "[The nurse] recognized that [the baby] wanted attention." A second nurse said,

I see the parents grow as much as he's [the baby] grown. I've helped them grow. They've gone from being overwhelmed, feeling anxiety about the equipment to the books to tell me about premature babies. They write questions to ask. They're assertive, not afraid. The baby comes first in their lives. I feel good about how far they've all come.

Knowing the patient enabled the nurse to "take into account his hearing loss, recognizing the patient's inability." Patients also acknowledged the nurse knew them: "She is buttoning my shirt." "She asks questions which seem pertinent to what's important to me."

Another nurse said: "You learn [sic] the baby, his reactions. There's a little individual there.... You get to learn the baby same as a friend, their likes and dislikes. Knowing the baby is like knowing the wires and how much stimulus he can handle."

To learn about the baby, one nurse said she, "focused on the parents and their needs.... [It was] taking care of the whole family. The parents are your major source."

A mother said, "She took care about the noises around the baby [because] she was sensitive to his needs." A nurse in a pediatric ICU said:

Initially that's all you see [the tubes and technology], maybe 6 months to a year ... then that becomes routine. The hard part is taking care of the patient. Physical care becomes mechanical; emotional caring is harder. You have control over the physical care, it becomes the easy part.

There's really no one way of approaching the family. There's the same approach to suctioning and IVs. Every family is different. I have 6 years experience here and I'm still learning emotional caring, emotional support.... It's knowing the family, being with them all the way through. For instance, a child was diagnosed with leukemia 2 $1/_2$ years ago. He relapsed 9 months ago, and was in and out, and then he died after Christmas.... I'll never forget the intensity of the emotional situation.

Concern

Concern is a word that many equate with caring itself. In this study, concern is a dimension of the relationship aspect of the communication of caring. "I am concerned about the client's reactions to her sister butting in.... I am listening to the family talk about their concerns [about Medicaid]." A mother stated, "She is concerned about foods and bathing, about making sure I'm not rushing them in their growing, about health, about crying." A patient noted, "When she talks to me, she thinks highly of me. I feel important that she is concerned." Another patient said, "She is showing concern about my own care, and concern about my headaches." A nurse commented, "I'm showing and saying my concern through the specific use of words." Another nurse explained, "I feel concern for this lady. I am caring in seeing her in so much pain. I am concerned about [how] she is suctioning her trach." And another nurse stated, "I am concerned about her health status."

SUMMARY

Building on premises of symbolic interactionism and the grounded-theory method, investigators have demonstrated that the basic social process of caring in nursing is communication in its irreducible aspects of content and relationship (Knowlden, 1985; Watzlawick et al., 1967). The aspect of nursing content—information—consisted of four major dimensions: physical care, health promotion, health assessment, and patient advocacy. The physical care dimension included properties of protecting, acknowledging physical limitations, and positioning. The health promotion dimension was primarily demonstrated through health teaching, although the safety element was also noted. The health assessment dimension included the properties of assessing physical and emotional health and assessing environment.

Assessment was conducted through examination, observation, and interview. Being a patient advocate, following up or following through, providing resources, going above and beyond, and collaborating were included in the patient advocacy dimension.

The nurse-patient relationship was indicated through five dimensions: dialogue; conveying progress and hope; attachment; knowing the patient, family, and significant others; and concern. Dialogue had the properties of verbal and nonverbal communication. Each of these properties had several sub-dimensions. The dimension conveying progress and hope had many characteristics. Among these were concentrating, building self-esteem, and being equal. The dimensions of attachment; knowing patients, families, and significant others; and concern, had no sub-dimensions.

Through the communication of caring in its aspects of content and relationship, nurses assist patients, families, and their significant others toward health or to a humane death. These caring practices by nurses are within the expectations and responsibilities that society generally and specifically holds for the discipline of nursing. Caring is the essence of nursing practice.

Chapter 4

CONDITIONS FOR CARING

Information concerning the conditions for caring—or not caring—were also identified. Among these were balance, definitions of caring, ethical concerns, lack of caring, holistic care, and institutional structures for caring for patients, families, and significant others.

BALANCE

Balance was a theme that originated mainly in the interviews with neonatal unit nurses. Nurses tried to balance the discomforts of the medical regimen, the parents' anxiety and the range of services involved "in treating babies." They tried to "determine when the baby needed more treatment and when she had had enough."

Some nurses said:

> [It] takes about a day to get control of the mechanical, to get a feeling for balance, that things will work out. You get a feeling of concern with the family's comfort. If they're uptight, you're in control. To create a balance, you talk more openly about things to get them prepared for the inevitable if the baby's to die. If you're comfortable, you allay the parents' anxiety. You take each patient and family as an individual.

One nurse stated that she would try to balance the discomforts with the parents' anxiety and the services involved. "I try to determine when [the patient and family] need more and when it's enough.... You get a feeling for balance, that things will work out."

One nurse's view of balance was particularly interesting:

> I see machines as extremities requiring lots of care and lots of technical skills. You have to find a balance between the technical and the nontechnical, yet you can't ignore the alarms or the IV fluids.... It's very difficult.

A nurse in a medical ICU described finding a balance when dealing with technology:

> Everyone provides emotional support during that time of crisis. But like now, with the balloon pump, we're not used to it. "I'll take care

of the balloon pump, if you'll take care of the patient." Now the main object of my caring is the machine which is taking care of keeping the patient's life going. You take care of the machine. You don't want to jeopardize that life. It's caring in that way.

Here two nurses are sharing the balance between caring and technology. The nurses realized that the demands of technology are equally challenged by the demands of caring for the person.

DEFINITIONS OF CARING

Definitions were determined after many interviews with patients or parents and with nurses. The definitions evolved as the videotapes were played back for home care participants' observations about caring and in the interviews in the ICU study. A mother of a baby in a neonatal ICU indicated caring was demonstrated when "One nurse picked him up. She loved him. She held him and rubbed his feet. She didn't care that he was attached to tubes."

An elderly home care patient who was recovering from a stroke stated, "The feeling bounces on me and bounces back again ... caring flows through the fingertips." A nurse working in a medical ICU indicated that "caring is being concerned, [truly concerned] about others' feelings, problems, situations, overall well-being." This same nurse described how she felt about herself when she'd been a caring nurse:

I felt good, happy with a sense of well-being. You've given something to someone else that you never could have—why you were where you were with that patient when he needed something and especially with the family when making life and death decisions.... Even if he doesn't pull through, I've done something else besides cure his disease. I see it also from the way the family is treating me differently.

As has been indicated elsewhere (Bishop & Scudder, 1991), the meaning of caring is revealed in the practices of caring.

ETHICAL CONCERNS

The narratives about ethical concerns were derived from the interviews with nurses, patients, and parents who participated in the ICU study. These concerns sometimes arose out of a sense of moral outrage participants felt about some aspect of their or their family member's care from health care providers. The concerns reflect Bishop and Scudder's (1990) definition of the moral sense as "fostering the well-being of patients" (p. 117) and as "for the good of the other" (p. 136). One neonatal intensive care nurse expressed it as follows:

As far as ethics go, ethical decisions lie more with physicians and parents than with nurses. Yet at times it's bothered me to do something to prolong life, it's going to end anyway. But it's the parents' baby and if they want those measures--[pauses]. If it [were] my baby, perhaps I'd act the same way.

She also indicated that "I always question the line between doing enough and doing too much.... When is there too much technology to keep someone alive longer than is meant to be." ·

A nurse in a medical ICU said:

What's hard is the patient who you have ambivalent feelings about as to the extent of technology. Then it takes all of you to make sure you care for the patient, not just do the task and leave. In this unit that happens frequently. We don't know when to stop and that makes it difficult to have the caring aspect.

The nurse in the pediatric surgical ICU caring for the patient with Rubenstein's taboid syndrome stated, "She's now on Levophed. I question why this is necessary. She's halfway over the hump in a critical situation."

Another nurse in a pediatric ICU discussed a baby with microcephaly:

Some parents are harder to talk to. They do not realize the seriousness of the illness. This baby has neuro problems. The parents think he is a normal baby who has bad lung disease. He's a bone. His sutures are closed. He eats one good feed a day with a nasogastric tube feeding at night. It's frustrating. As you know, he's hungry.... He vomits if he eats too much.... No one's telling the family the truth. Most kids aren't on steroids and he is.... If he's not going to die, I don't know how much more we're going to do. It's tragic. He's content with his mother.

A neonatal ICU nurse cried as she recounted a situation with "a baby who was terminal. The family knew it and accepted it. But the docs continued to draw blood. I argued with them, and then.... Finally the docs left him alone."

In this situation the nurse's ethical concern extended to the baby's dying:

When it came time for him to come off the vent, the parents decided not to be here. I came in even though it was my day off and held him to die. The thought of him dying without anyone who knew him tore me apart. It wasn't fair.

LACK OF CARING

Instances of the lack of caring were discussed by some participants. For example, a mother whose son had been moved from the neonatal intensive care unit to the pediatric ICU commented on the lack of caring by a primary nurse. What the mother says is not solely in response to the lack of caring by the nurse.

Some can take care of but not know how to care.... Some wouldn't understand, but most do. I'd just ask them to put themselves in your position.... It's the simple things. There's a difference in giving a baby a bath. Don't just stick the baby under the faucet, but gently put the baby in the water and hold him gently in a towel.

In the beginning, I had a different primary and I asked to have her removed. It's not that she was doing anything wrong. She just lacked, I guess, a bedside manner ... I did not want primary care from just any person. I did not want poor handling or a lack of warmth.

The mother pleaded for the well-being of her son; as a result, he received care that fostered his growth.

HOLISTIC CARE

The narratives concerning holistic care came from an elderly patient in the home-care study and from nurses in the ICU study. The patient, ill with chronic obstructive pulmonary disease, said:

The questions she asks shows she's alert and wants to learn about me.... She's interested in the emotional part of patients like when she wants to know why I get shaky and upset.... She's interested in the whole patient, not just pains and aches. Emotions tell so much about what's real.

A nurse who had worked in a neonatal ICU for 6 years stated, "There's really no [one] way of approaching each family. There's the same approach to suctioning and IVs, but every family is different." Holistic care for one neonatal ICU nurse meant understanding the parents' religion and using that knowledge to be an advocate for the baby's rights as she interpreted the parents' position to other health care professionals.

INSTITUTIONAL STRUCTURES FOR CARING

In some interviews in the ICU study, participants discussed policies that made caring possible. One participant said, "You make accommodations for the quad at home to visit." A nurse in the pediatric ICU said:

The playroom is staffed. Parents can visit at any time. Volunteers come in to provide cuddling. There's adequate staffing—you care for no more than three children in here. We allow siblings to visit the unit. There's always a nurse in the room.

Some neonatal and pediatric ICUs had provision for a cuddler program. In these units, volunteers are "trained to cuddle babies who need cuddling, extra care, and attention.... A baby on a vent who needs stroking and sometimes feeding and changing.... There are rooms for family visiting, but we need a sibling room."

One mother whose baby had been in the neonatal ICU said, "The cuddler program was very good. It's important for babies to get attention and get held. They hold and rock the babies. That makes a big difference." Another mother stated that in the neonatal ICU the nurses, "primaries, were on 12-hour shifts and that helped the babies." She went on to say that once her son graduated to the pedi ICU, "There was not as much warmth. They were understaffed and not able to do as much ... I thought it would be better in pedi. There he was, starting to be a baby, but still with life and death needs."

Elaine's mother stated that the nurses "let me know to call any time. I rarely talked to the night nurses, but at times I would call."

In contrast there were policies which were deemed necessary in order to care for people in critical situations but which excluded families. A nurse working in a cardiac care unit stated,

There is the harshness of the unit, of the staff as a group toward the families when the patients first come in. They've got to wait in the waiting room. In time it [the focus] turns back to the family, but [the initial pushing away] may seem harsh to them. It's hard initially to even it out, as the patient then is the priority. There seems no other way to do it. Later we can explain it to them. Sometimes I'll go explain what's going on with the patient if it's someone else's patient. That seems to help.

And in the neonatal ICU a nurse noted that the procedures initiated following the birth of the infant, and which excluded parents, must seem uncaring however necessary they are. "After a baby is born, and admitted to the unit, the father is not allowed to come in until after the lines are started, the baby's intubated, and the vent's on."

Some nurses and parents recognized the importance of charting. "It's important to do the documenting accurately," one nurse stated. Elaine's mother noted that the nurses "had a category for when parents come in, and it was noted on the chart." Another mother commented about the importance of charting her son's progress, and nurses noted the significance of keeping care plans up to date.

Only one person, a patient—the 40-year-old man who had had a heart attack—commented on the discrepancies in salary paid to physicians and nurses:

I don't think I overestimate the difficulty of the job ... the separation in salary and the hierarchical order for the doctors is greatly exaggerated. Hospitals should create many positions of grades between [the nurses] and the doctors, so that they reach the same salary limits.

In the home-care study both patients and nurses noted that when an agency restructured districts, these arbitrary decisions broke long-term nurse-patient relationships. Patients missed their nurses, felt abandoned, and resented having to start anew with another nurse. Nurses, too, missed patients and regretted that some therapeutic nursing actions had to be discontinued. In these instances they believed their nursing services were devalued.

SUMMARY

This chapter has presented some conditions for caring in nursing. These conditions indicate that caring is more than a mere behavior between nurse and patient. They indicate that caring requires that the expectations, norms, and values of both the American culture and the nursing profession be reflected in organizational policies and practices.

Chapter 5

CONCLUSIONS

In this monograph, I have presented the synthesis of two grounded-theory studies of caring in the practice of nursing. The content of the synthesis was drawn from interviews with nurses, patients, patients' families and significant others in home and intensive-care settings.

Participants in the studies consisted of 45 patients, parents, and significant others and 39 nurses. The majority of patients were over age 40 (*n*=31) and had completed high school or higher education. Their diagnoses varied. Most nurses were between 21 and 39 years of age (*n*=33). Most had a baccalaureate degree (*n*=27). Nurses encountered their patients in homes and clinics, and in medical, neonatal, pediatric, and surgical ICUs. This resulting monograph is focused on the meanings of caring in nursing situations. The findings are significant in that no other researchers of caring by nurses have discussed the centrality of communication in conveying caring as the essence of nursing.

The findings from the synthesis indicate that caring in nursing is interpersonal communication between the nurse and the patient, family, and significant others. Caring communication consists of the irreducible aspects of content and relationship (Watzlawick et al., 1967). Nursing content is demonstrated in four categories: physical care, health promotion, health assessment, and patient advocacy. The relationship aspect is conveyed through five categories: dialogue; conveying progress and hope; attachment; knowing the patient, family, and significant others; and concern (Figure 5.1). Neither aspect is present without the other in any communication of caring in nursing.

This is a significant finding in that it is through communication that caring, the essence of nursing, is conveyed. Caring is a human trait. Some actions defined as relationship in this study are common everyday actions of one human to another. However, it is the content aspect of nurse caring that makes the caring of nursing practice specific to the discipline of nursing. Caring by nurses is both like and unlike caring as being human. It is like caring as being human in that the relationship is a human trait. It is unlike caring in being human in that the content matter of the discipline of nursing is learned and then enacted as caring relationships

Figure 5.1 Synthesized Model of the Communication of Caring in Nursing

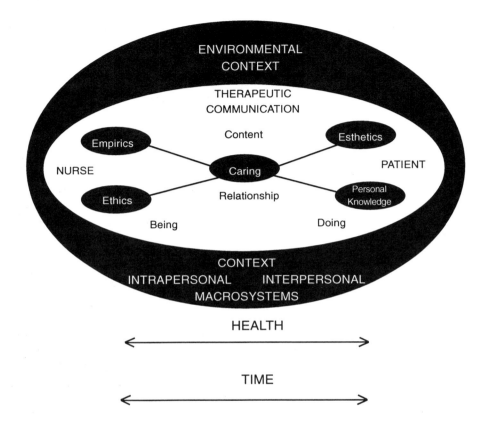

in the practice of the nurse. Knowledge of health and illness; knowledge of human responses to illness; knowledge of human anatomy, physiology, psychology, sociology, history; and the inseparable relationship aspect of being human, all contribute to the irreducibility of the communication of caring in nursing practice.

The aspect of relationship is studied and learned as well. It is learned by growing up in a family, a community, and a culture. It is also learned through the educational, programmatic, political, and socialization practices of the nursing curriculum and the mission of the college, and through the employing organizations and agencies of the larger society.

Grounded-theory investigators explore fundamental psychosocial and structural processes that constitute human relationships. Grounded-theory practitioners use field-research methods to identify and describe actions in naturalistic settings. It provides an orderly guide for theory development. As stated earlier, grounded theory is drawn from symbolic interactionism and articulates its basic premises. Researchers interpret the data from the field to discover the meaning, which results in the grounded theory. In this study, I look at the process of being a caring nurse. Thus, it is an ontological study of the nature of being a nurse (Roach, 1984).

THE PRACTICE OF CARING

The communication of caring by nurses occurs through their practices—their actions. Such practices are derived from a thorough knowledge of the patient by a nurse who may use the nursing process but who also understands that patients are more than nursing care plans—a nurse who thinks about patients and their situations holistically and humanely. Caring nurses are in connection with their patients (Marcel, 1951) and recognize that through encounter with patients they are able to move from the objective "It-world" to the world of relation (Buber, 1970).

Patients in these studies know this connection through their participation in care. They were able to recall and to recapture in interviews caring and noncaring by nurses. They were active participants in their getting better. In general, caring in nursing is not one-sided, but experienced reciprocally by nurses and patients.

The communication of caring by nurses is a process that occurs through the steadfastness of the nurses' caring for or caring about patients, families, or significant others in situations in which they need nursing care. The irreducibility of content and relationship in communicating caring is demonstrated through the nurses' actions. Nursing content actions do not occur without simultaneous relationship actions. Relationship aspects of the communication of caring appear to exist alongside the content aspects of nursing practice. A neonatal intensive care nurse, while listening to a mother struggling with her infant's experience with the side effects with a drug, taught the mother how to advocate for her child's needs, supported her in her actions, and simultaneously built her self-esteem. The nurse went beyond expectations in this situation because the baby had already been discharged. She displayed attachment and concern as well as a caring connectedness.

Nurses' communication of caring occurs during their practice. As such, they are social acts. They are to be understood in the social context of the nursing situation. Nurses' practices are caring acts when "view[ed] ... from the standpoint of rights, obligations, and expectations involved in that situation" (Blumer, 1969, p. 178). The communication of caring is also to be understood as an ethic of care—that is, of responsibility, connection, and relationships (Tronto, 1987).

Some conditions for caring were also discovered. Nurses talked about searching for balance in their practice between the needs of patients and those of the medical regimen. Participants, both patients and nurses, noted how norms and values are reflected in organizations' policies, practices, and structures. These conditions and structures affect the way caring and noncaring nursing occurs.

IMPLICATIONS

This study reflects several implications for nurse caring in education, practice, research, and the profession. Ultimately, the goal of communicating caring in nursing is caring about the health of patients or for their right to die humanely.

EDUCATION

For nurses, learning about caring is initiated in their education. As Leininger (1986) indicated,

> Students need to be taught early in their programs of study about the concepts of generic and professional care and how they are used to give nursing care. They need to discover that care is literally in their hands by what they know, see, and do (p. 4).

Curricula, which enable teacher and practitioner role modeling, provide opportunities for learning caring among students, teachers, and practitioners. An educational process that demonstrates the contributions of the humanities, and natural and social sciences to the development of therapeutic nursing actions advances the development of caring practitioners (Figure 6.1). How students are taught influences how they learn to care. A nurse educator who provides case studies, stories, or videotapes of situations with patients, and then explicates the caring actions used grounds the content of nursing practice in the context of the patient situation. This is one way the learning of nurse caring occurs.

PRACTICE

Nurses in clinical practice are already in a patient situation, and nurse caring is shaped by the context of their patients' lives. From knowledge of both the content of nursing and of the relationship aspects of being human, their nursing practice becomes a caring practice. The policies and structures of the practice setting also shape nurse caring. In practice settings in which a study of the meaning of caring has been undertaken, conditions and structures for caring will have been developed (Valentine, 1991).

The present research demonstrates that nurses understand integrating caring with the use of technology, but contextual pressures may interfere with the thoughtful reflection required to communicate that caring. One difficulty in contemporary nursing practice is the erosion of conditions for such reflection. Economic and fiscal pressures sometimes lead to a belief that people do not matter.

RESEARCH

In the last decade, many studies about caring in nursing have been completed. However, as Morse and her colleagues (1991) noted, few researchers have investigated the activities and experiences of nurse caring with families, groups, and communities. Studies are needed that show how the knowledge about caring is shaping curricula and thus practice. Continuing studies about how caring is practiced in institutions and agencies using managed care are needed. Extensive theory development about caring and its use in education and practice are critical if nursing is to continue to claim that caring is the essence of nursing.

THE PROFESSION

Through studies, and through exposure to economics, institutions, organizations, and politics—nurses can determine if the caring that is taught in curricula is internalized and carried out. The profession, through its organizations, then acts through policy statements to ensure that nursing care and health care reflect the values and concerns of the profession. Professional organizations which take and defend stances that reflect what has been valued in the practice of nursing, by both nurses and society, energize nurses through their acts of commitment to caring about the profession.

CONCLUSION

The communication of caring in nursing occurs in a dialogue with patients, families, and significant others to promote and maintain health. Consisting of the two irreducible aspects of communication, content, and relationship, caring is demonstrated through the therapeutic nursing actions of conveying progress and hope; dialogue; teaching about health; assessing health; acting as a patient advocate; being attached; knowing the patient, family, and significant others; being concerned; and providing physical care. These findings are significant in that they demonstrate the holistic nature of caring in nursing practice. Caring is the essence, the core of nursing practice (Leininger, 1977).

Chapter 6

THE THEORY OF
CARING IN NURSING

In this chapter, an analysis and evaluation of the theory of communication of caring in nursing will be presented. The format for the analysis
and evaluation was drawn from Fawcett (1992, 1993) and Meleis (1991).
The analysis gives the opportunity to present the theory in the formal
manner of a set of concepts and propositions, and to identify its scope
and context. The evaluation gives the opportunity to determine the extent to which the theory meets the context of significance. Fawcett (1992,
1993) notes that theory scope, context, and content; conceptual-theoreti-
cal-empirical, structure; diagram(s); the relationship between theory and
research; significance; internal consistency; parsimony; testability; operational, empirical, and pragmatic adequacy are all criteria to be considered.
Meleis (1991) takes into account the structural and functional components and raises many cogent questions concerning theory analysis and
evaluation. Fawcett's criteria will be followed generally with consideration
given to Meleis' concerns.

ANALYSIS

SCOPE OF THE THEORY

This middle-range theory of the communication of caring in nursing is
focused on interpersonal relationships among nurses, patients, and significant others who are in need of nursing. Communication of caring in
nursing occurs in a dialogue with patients, families, and significant others
to promote and maintain health or have a humane death. Consisting of
the two irreducible aspects of communication—content and relationship—
caring is conveyed through the therapeutic nursing actions of conveying
progress and hope; dialogue; teaching about health; assessing health; acting as a patient advocate; being attached; knowing the patient, family,
and significant others; being concerned; and providing physical care.

The theory indicates how caring is provided in nursing situations, generated from grounded-theory research, and is both descriptive and ex-

planatory. Evaluation of the theory reveals its significance for holistic caring in nursing practice.

The scope of the theory is broad in that it focuses on how caring is provided by nurses to patients and families in two diverse settings: home care and hospital ICUs. Thus it can be useful in a variety of nursing situations. From the theory, nurses in practice and education can envision and then enact how the nursing content and the relationship between nurses and care receivers work together in providing care. The importance of environments of all sorts is acknowledged in the theory.

The goal of nursing is providing care intended to help the return to health or the humane death of patients. Problems addressed by the theory involve people who need nursing in health-illness situations.

Nursing therapeutics are determined by these situations encountered by nurses and their clients—and include therapeutic use of self, communication techniques, deliberate actions of teaching, physical care, safety, positioning, assessing, and so on.

Decision-making is mutually accomplished among nurses, patients, and families but depends on the situation. Nurses play many roles in the course of communicating caring including teacher, caregiver, care manager, collaborator, technician, advocate, and assessor. The goal of studying the theory is to understand how nurses communicate caring to patients, families, and significant others. It provides knowledge for the communication of caring in nursing.

CONTEXT OF THE THEORY

Metaparadigm Concepts

The theory encompasses all the metaparadigm concepts—person, nursing, environment, and health. Within the theory of the communication of caring in nursing,

1. Person refers to humans as individuals or groups.

2. Nursing refers to professional nursing care (caring) ... formal and cognitively learned professional care knowledge and practice skills obtained through educational institutions that are used to provide assistive, supportive, enabling, or facilitative acts to or for another individual or group in order to improve a human health condition (or well-being), disability, lifeway, or to work with dying clients (Leininger, in Fawcett, 1993, p. 58).

The view of nursing is that of an interactional process between humans in situations in which one partner needs nursing, and the other provides it.

This researcher concurs with Watson (1990) that caring should be a central concept in the nursing metaparadigm; the thing—nursing—cannot be a member of itself. The word caring should replace the word nursing in the metaparadigm.

3. Environmental context "refers to the totality of an event, situation, or particular experiences that give meaning to human expressions, interpretations, and social interactions in particular physical, ecological, sociopolitical, or cultural settings" (Leininger, in Fawcett, 1993, p. 57).
4. Health is a state of well-being and balance in one's life. Illness is a state of unbalance, unhealthiness.

Philosophic Claims

The work has been strongly influenced by Symbolic Interactionism, Leininger's and Watson's theories of caring, qualitative research perspectives, humanistic values and ideals, and the importance of connectedness between people.

Philosophic Assumptions

1. Caring is the essence of humans surviving; caring is the essence of nursing.
2. "Tacit knowledge [is] the base on which the human ... builds many of the insights that ... eventually develop" (Lincoln & Guba, 1985, p. 198).
3. Researcher and participants were equal partners in coming to understand caring in nursing. They were valued and respected equally. This is true also of the nurse-patient-family relationship.
4. Self-reflexivity is an important human characteristic.
5. Meaning is individually constructed.

Antecedent Knowledge

The theory has been shaped by my personal values concerning life and relationships, through dialogue, reading widely, thinking, and curiosity about people and how they live. Other pertinent knowledge comes out of my experience as a psychiatric nurse with background in psychology, psychiatry, sociology, anthropology, and world literature based on undergraduate majors in nursing and English and minors in sociology and French; and as nurse educator and researcher with wide reading in philosophy, education, and scientific methodology. These have all contributed to the theory's development.

CONTENT OF THE THEORY

Concepts

From this grounded-theory research concerning caring in nursing, a theory emerged. The main constructs of the theory are caring, communication, and the irreducible communication aspects of content and relationship. Caring in nursing occurs through communication of nursing content and the relationship among nurses, patients, families, and significant others. Caring communication is complex and multidimensional.

Any communication always has a content aspect and a relationship aspect. Communication refers to "a process by which information is exchanged between individuals through a common system of symbols, signs, or behavior" (Webster 10th edition, 1995, p. 233). Content refers to the information contained in the communication. In the theory, content includes the four dimensions of physical care, health promotion, health assessment, and patient advocacy (see Table 6.1 for definitions).

Table 6.1 Constitutive Definitions for the Dimensions of the Theory	
Dimension	Constitutive Definition
Attachment	A theme of relationship that illustrates the mutuality among nurses, patients, families, and significant others.
Concern	A theme of relationship frequently used by the discipline of nursing to define caring itself. In the theory, concern means that the situation of the patient, family, and significant others matters.
Conveying Progress & Hope	A theme of relationship that reflects the actions nurses take to let patients know that they are important in and of themselves, and considered equal as human beings.
Dialogue	A theme of relationship that describes communicating caring through speech and other nonverbal communication.
Health Assessment	A theme of content that describes nurses' activities in overseeing and promoting patients' health.
Health Promotion	A theme of content that is characterized essentially by health teaching, and is considered critical to patients' well-being and healing.
Knowing the Patient, Significant Others	A theme that describes the importance of a family, patient's history and present, and circumstances to the provision of care.
Patient Advocacy	A theme of content that refers to nursing actions which confirm to patients their worth.
Physical Care	A theme of content that encompasses the hands-on aspect of nursing care and derives its meaning from its subthemes.

Relationship refers to the metacommunication about the communication, is virtually all nonverbal, and includes the nature of the relationship, action cues, and vocal cues present in the context of the interaction. In the theory, relationship includes the five dimensions of dialogue; conveying progress and hope; attachment; knowing the patient, family and significant others; and concern (see Table 6.1 for definitions).

As one views these definitions of the content and relationship aspects of the communication of caring in nursing, it must always be remembered that the aspects are irreducible. Caring in nursing is comprised of the presence of at least one content aspect with at least one relationship aspect. Caring in nursing is not expressed only by demonstrating concern. Caring in nursing is expressed by communicating concern while doing health assessment or health teaching. It is expressed in physical care along with gentle touching. Patient advocacy occurs with knowing patients, families, and significant others.

Meta-themes, conditions for communicating caring in nursing, were also identified: balance, personal definitions of caring, ethical concerns, nursing practice experience, holistic care, instances of not caring, and institutional structures for caring for patients, families, and/or significant others.

Propositions

1. Caring is essential for human survival. Caring in nursing is essential for patients' return to health or humane death.
2. The theory's constructs are irreducible and represent a holistic view of the nurse-patient relationship including family and significant others. Irreducibility indicates that communications among nurse-patient-family are always composed of content and relationship. Communication of caring cannot be transformed to a simpler condition. The importance of the ongoing interacting whole of nurse, patient, family, and environment—holism—is recognized.
3. Nursing actions bring restoration in the patient's health and well-being or assist in a humane death. In the theory, the nursing actions which comprise the irreducible content and relationship aspects are symbolic in conveying the meaning of the communication of caring in nursing.
4. Despite the continued threat of technology and bureaucratization, nurses continue to provide caring nursing to humans in need. The communication of caring in nursing mitigates the domination of technology through focus on the patient as a person, a whole subject for care, not as an object to be done to. Communication of caring in nursing recognizes that patients are individuals with histories and futures and with their own understandings and meanings for their health situations.

CONCEPTUAL-THEORETICAL-EMPIRICAL STRUCTURE

The conceptual structure is derived from the philosophies of symbolic interactionism and caring, and the theories of communication and nurse caring. The constant comparative method of grounded theory (Glaser & Strauss, 1967), a qualitative research method derived from symbolic interactionism, was utilized for data analysis, interpretation, and writing the theory. Figures 5.1 and 6.1 were constructed to display the irreducibility of the two aspects of communication—content and relationship—and their nine dimensions. The diagrams depict the holistic nature of the communication of caring in nursing. They also depict the holistic nature of nursing practice.

Figure 6.1 The Communication of Caring in Nursing (Model 2)

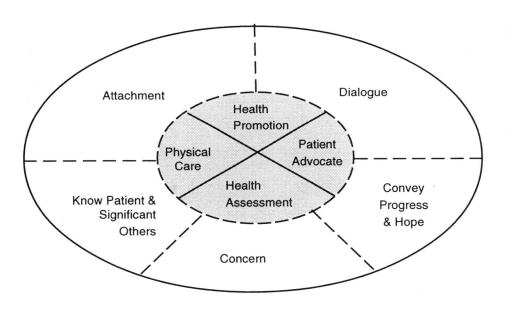

Inner Circle = Content
Outer Circle = Relationship

EVALUATION

SIGNIFICANCE

The significance of a theory lies in its importance to the discipline of nursing. Fawcett (1992) indicated that the criterion of significance "is met when the metaparadigmatic, philosophic, and paradigmatic origins of the theory are explicit; when the adjunctive knowledge is cited; and when the special contributions made by the theory are identified" (p. 42). The metaparadigmatic, philosophic, and paradigmatic origins of the theory have been documented above. The adjunctive knowledge is specified. The special contribution of understanding caring in nursing as interpersonal communication in its irreducible aspects of content and relationship is indicated.

INTERNAL CONSISTENCE

The criterion of internal consistency is met. The philosophic claims, conceptual model, and theory are congruent. The communication of caring in nursing is described in its two irreducible aspects with their nine dimensions. The concepts reflect semantic clarity in that they are not redundant. The concepts also reflect semantic consistency, because definitions of concepts as constructs and dimensions remain constant throughout the monograph. The propositions demonstrate structural consistency in the logical manner of their relationships.

PARSIMONY

Formal analysis and evaluation of the theory of the communication of caring in nursing indicates that the criterion of parsimony is met. The communication of caring is a single construct with two irreducible aspects and nine dimensions. Thus, it is efficiently expressed without oversimplification.

TESTABILITY

Although qualitative research does not emphasize replicability, it is possible to replicate the studies to test the theory. Utilizing symbolic interactionism and caring for the philosophic and conceptual foundation, a grounded-theory methodology could again be used with the same research question in settings other than those used by this researcher. Such research could further establish the trustworthiness and confirmability of the interpretation of the findings which led to the theory, and expand its meaning for the discipline of nursing (Lincoln & Guba, 1985).

OPERATIONAL, EMPIRICAL, AND PRAGMATIC ADEQUACY

The research design, which led to the theory of the communication of caring in nursing, meets the criterion of operational adequacy. The nurse and patient or parent participants in the studies were partners in the nursing situations. Each had experienced the events of the situation and was able to comment upon those events. The description of the constant comparative method utilized in grounded-theory methodology is in keeping with that reported by Glaser & Strauss (1967) and others.

The criterion of empirical adequacy as a measure of the degree of confidence in the "truth" of the theory was met by having findings confirmed by participants via "member checks," by a panel of nurse experts, and by professional colleagues and the lay public via formal presentations of the theory.

Pragmatic adequacy has been achieved through the use of the theory as one dimension in framing a professional nursing education curriculum. The theory has not been formally used in practice settings.

CONCLUSION

The theory contributes significantly to knowledge for the discipline of nursing. It is the first published theory that shows both nurse and patient contributions to the nurse-patient situation as well as to the research undertaking. It is also the first to indicate how essential communication is in the matter of restoring a patient to health or helping them have a humane death. Humans cannot *not* communicate, just as they cannot not care. Fawcett's (1992, 1993) and Meleis' (1991) frameworks of theory analysis and evaluation have been used to substantiate the theory of caring in nursing.

References

Andrews, L.W., Daniels, B., & Hull, A.G. (1996). Nurse caring behaviors: comparing five to define perceptions. *Ostomy/Wound Management, 42*(5), 28-37.

Benner, P. (1984). *From novice to expert.* CA: Addison-Wesley.

Benner, P., & Wrubel, J. (1989). *The primacy of caring.* CA: Addison-Wesley.

Benoliel, J.Q. (1996). Grounded theory and nursing knowledge. *Qualitative Health Research, 6*(3), 406-428.

Berger, M.M. (1978). *Videotape techniques in psychiatric training and treatment.* NY: Bruner-Mazel.

Bevis, E.O. (1981). Caring: A life force. In M. Leininger (Ed.), *Caring: An essential human need.* Thorofare, NJ: Chas. B. Slack.

Bevis, E.O. (1982). *Curriculum building in nursing,* (3rd ed.). St. Louis, MO: C.V. Mosby.

Bishop, A.H., & Scudder, Jr., J.R. (1990). *The practical, moral, and personal sense of nursing.* Albany, NY: SUNY Press.

Bishop, A.H., & Scudder, Jr., J.R. (1991). *Nursing: The practice of caring.* NY: National League for Nursing Press.

Blumer, H. (1967). Society as symbolic interaction. In J.G. Manis & B.N. Meltzer (Eds.), *Symbolic Interaction.* Boston: Allyn & Bacon.

Blumer, H. (1969). *Symbolic Interactionism.* Englewood Cliffs, NJ: Prentice-Hall.

Bowers, B.J. (1988). Grounded Theory. In B. Sarter, *Paths to knowledge.* NY: National League for Nursing.

Buber, M. (1970). *I and Thou.* (W. Kaufmann, Translator). NY: Charles Scribner's Sons.

Carper, B.A. (1979). The ethics of caring. *Advances in Nursing Science, 1*(3), 11-19.

Chenitz, W.C., & Swanson, J.M. (1986). *From practice to grounded theory.* CA: Addison-Wesley Publishing.

Conway, M. (1978). Theoretical approaches to the study of role. In M.E. Hardy, & M. Conway, *Role theory: Perspectives for health professionals.* NY: Appleton Century Crofts.

Corbin, J. (1986). Qualitative data analysis for grounded theory. In W.C. Chenitz & J.M. Swanson, *From practice to grounded theory.* CA: Addison-Wesley Publishing.

Donaldson, S.K., & Crowley, D. (1978). The discipline of nursing. *Nursing Outlook, 26*(2), 113-120.

Drew, N. (1986). Exclusion and confirmation. *Image: Journal of Nursing Scholarship, 18*(2): 39-43.

Fawcett, J. (1993). *Analysis and evaluation of nursing theories.* Philadelphia: F.A. Davis.

Fawcett, J., & Downs, F.S. (1992). *The relationship of theory and research.* Philadelphia: F.A. Davis.

Glaser, B.G. (1978). *Theoretical sensitivity.* Mill Valley, CA: The Sociology Press.

Glaser, B.G., & Strauss, A. (1967). *The discovery of grounded theory.* NY: Aldine Publishing.

Hardy, M.E. (1988). Perspectives on science. *Role theory perspectives for health professionals* (2nd ed.). NY: Appleton & Lange.

Hardy, M.E., & Hardy, W.L. (1988). Development of scientific knowledge. In M.E. Hardy & M. Conway, *Role theory perspectives for health professionals* (2nd ed.). NY: Appleton & Lange.

Hutchinson, S. (1986). Grounded theory: the method. In P.L. Munhall & C.J. Oiler, *Nursing Research: A qualitative perspective.* Norwalk, CT: Appleton-Century-Crofts.

Joas, H. (1985). *G.H. Mead: A Contemporary Re-examination of his Thought.* (R. Meyer, Translator). Cambridge, MA: The MIT Press.

Kaplan, A. (1964). *The conduct of inquiry.* NY: Harper & Row.

Knowlden, V. (1983). *Caring in nursing: Post-clinical conferences.* Paper presented at the 6th National Caring Conference, University of Texas—Tyler.

Knowlden, V. (1985). *The meaning of caring in the nursing role.* Ann Arbor, MI: University Microfilms International.

Knowlden, V. (1988). *Final report to the Lindbergh Foundation* (unpublished paper).

Kolb, T. (1978). Preface. In M.M. Berger, *Videotape techniques in psychiatric training and treatment.* NY: Bruner-Mazel.

Kools, S., McCarthy, M., Durham, R., & Robrecht, L. (1996). Dimensional analysis: Broadening the conception of grounded theory. *Qualitative Health Research, 6*(3), 312-330.

Lea, A., & Watson, R. (1996). Caring research and concepts: A selected review of the literature. *Journal of Clinical Nursing, 5*(2), 71-77.

Leininger, M. (1977). Caring: The essence & central focus of nursing. *Nursing Research Reports, 12*(1), 2,14.

Leininger, M. (1980). Caring: A central focus of nursing and health care services. *Nursing & Health Care, 1*(3), 135.

Leininger, M. (1986). Care facilitation and resistance: Factors in the culture of nursing. *Topics in Clinical Nursing, 8*(2), 1-12.

Lincoln, Y.S., & Guba, E.G. (1985). *Naturalistic inquiry.* CA: Sage Publications.

Lowenburg, J.S. (1993). Interpretive research methodology: broadening the dialogue. *Advances in Nursing Science,* 16(2), 57-69.

Marcel, G. (1951). *Mystery of being: Faith & reality,* Vol. II. (R. Hague, Translator). South Bend, IN: Regnery/Gateway, Inc.

May, K.A. (1986). Writing and evaluating the grounded theory research report. In W.C. Chenitz & J.M. Swanson, *From practice to grounded theory.* CA: Addison-Wesley.

Mayeroff, M. (1971). *On Caring.* NY: Harper & Row.

Mead, G.H. (1934). *Mind, self and society.* C.W. Morris (Ed.). Chicago: University of Chicago Press.

Mead, G.H. (1956). *The Social psychology of G.H. Mead.* A. Strauss (Ed.). Chicago: University of Chicago Press.

Meleis, A.I. (1991). *Theoretical Nursing, 2nd ed.,* Philadelphia: J.B. Lippincott.

Merriam Webster's Collegiate Dictionary, 10th ed. (1995). Springfield, MA: G.C. Merriam Co.

Meyer, G.R. (1960). *Tenderness & technique: Nursing values in transition.* Los Angeles, CA: Institute of Industrial Relations.

Morse, J.M., Solberg, S., Neander, W.L., Bottorff, J.L., & Johnson, J.L. (1990). Concepts of caring and caring as a concept. *Advances in Nursing Science, 13*(1), 1-14.

Morse, J.M., Bottorff, J., Neander, W., & Solberg, S. (1991). Comparative analysis of conceptualizations and theories of caring. *Image: Journal of Nursing Scholarship, 23*(2), 119-126.

Noblit, G.W., & Hare, R.D. (1988). *Meta-Ethnography: Synthesizing qualitative studies.* Beverly Hills, CA: Sage Publications.

Polanyi, M. & Prosch, H. (1975). *Meaning.* Chicago: University of Chicago Press.

Prus, R. (1996). *Symbolic interactionism & ethnographic research.* NY: State University of New York Press.

Roach, S. (1984). *Caring: the human mode of being, implications for nursing.* Toronto: University of Toronto Faculty of Nursing.

Shiber, S., & Larson, E. (1991). Evaluating the quality of caring: structure, process, and outcome. *Holistic Nursing Practice, 5*(3), 57-66.

Stern, P.N. (1980). Grounded theory methodology: Its uses and processes. *Image: Journal of Nursing Scholarship, 12,* 20-23.

Stuart, G.W., & Sundeen, S.J. (1983). *Principles & practice of psychiatric nursing.* St. Louis, MO: C. V. Mosby.

Swanson, K.M. (1990). Providing care in the NICU: Sometimes an act of love. *Advances in Nursing Science, 13*(1), 60-73.

Swanson, K.M. (1991). Empirical development of a middle range theory of caring. *Nursing Research, 40*(3), 161-166.

Swanson, K.M. (1993). Nursing as informed caring for the well-being of others. *Image: Journal of Nursing Scholarship, 25*(4), 352-357.

Swanson-Kauffmann, K.M. (1986). Caring in the instance of unexpected early pregnancy loss. *Topics in Clinical Nursing, 8*(2), 37-46.

Tronto, J. (1987). Beyond gender difference to a theory of care. *Signs, 12*(4), 644-663.

Valentine, K. (1988). History, analysis, and application of the carative tradition in health and nursing, *Journal of the New York State Nurses Association, 19*(4), 4-9.

Valentine, K. (1989a). Caring is more than kindness; modeling its complexities. *Journal of Nursing Administration, 19*(11), 28-35.

Valentine, K. (1989b). A pragmatic research based justification for the value of caring. Paper presented at the Conn. State Nurses Association, Fall 1989.

Valentine, K. (1989c). The value of caring nurses: Implications for patient satisfaction, quality of care and cost. Paper presented at the Conn. State Nurses Association, Fall 1989.

Valentine, K.L. (1991). Comprehensive assessment of caring and its relationship to outcome measures. *Journal of Nursing Quality Assurance, 5*(2), 59-68.

Valentine, K. (1992). Strategic planning for professional practice. *Journal of Nursing Care Quality, 6*(3), 1-12.

Warren, L.D. (1988). Review and synthesis of nine nursing studies on care and caring. *Journal of the New York State Nurses Assoc., 19(4)*, 10-16

Watson, J. (1979). *Nursing: The philosophy and science of caring.* Boston, MA: Little Brown.

Watson, J. (1985). *Nursing: human science and human care.* CT: Appleton-Century-Crofts.

Watson, J. (1988). New dimensions in human caring theory. *Nursing Science Quarterly 1,* 175-181.

Watson, J. (1990). Caring knowledge and informed moral passion. *Advances in Nursing Science, 13*(1), 15-24.

Watzlawick, P., Beavin, J.H., & Jackson, D. (1967). *Pragmatics of human communication.* NY: W.W. Norton.

Wilson, A.S. (1989). Research in Nursing, 2nd ed., CA: Addison-Wesley.

Wolf, Z.R., Giardino, E.R., Osborne, P.A., & Ambrose, M.S. (1994). Dimensions of nurse caring. *Image: Journal of Nursing Scholarship, 26*(2), 107-111.